PLANT-BASED COOKBOOK FOR MEN

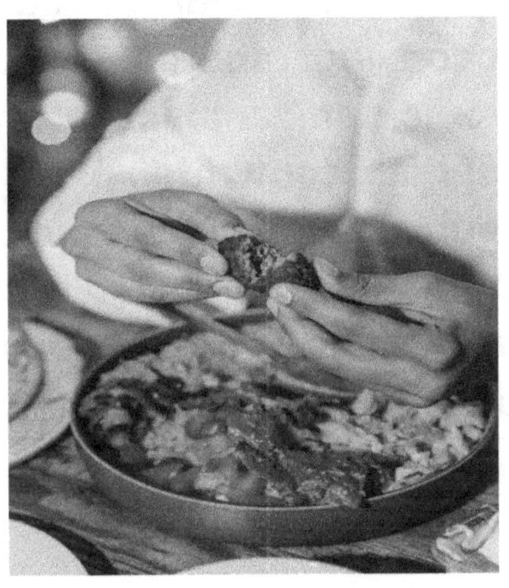

"Fueling Strength: A Bold Approach to Plant-Based Living for Men, With Over 30 Delicious And Healthy Recipe"

EMMA LYNCH

TABLE OF CONTENTS

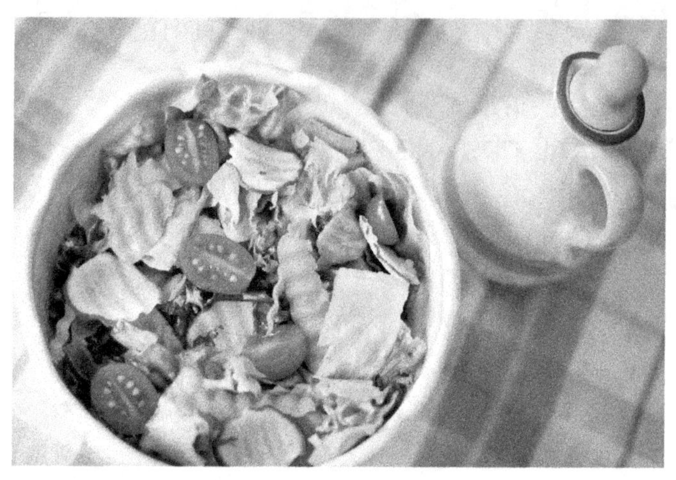

INTRODUCTION

In a world saturated with fads and diets, here's a proclamation: real strength and vitality begin in the kitchen. Imagine a culinary voyage where your plate isn't just a canvas for flavor but a compass guiding you to peak performance. What if I told you that the choice between a fork and a dumbbell isn't as binary as it seems?

Have you ever felt the pulsating energy of wholesome ingredients infusing life into your body? Can the sizzle of a pan tell a story of transformation, not just of food but of self? Picture this: a man navigating the realm of plant-based eating, not as a sacrifice but as an empowering journey.

Join me on an odyssey through these pages, where each recipe is a chapter, and every dish is a step towards a healthier, more vibrant you. This isn't just a cookbook; it's a narrative—a story of strength, flavor, and the inexorable connection between the fuel you choose and the man you become.

BENEFITS OF PLANT-BASED EATING

Plant-based eating offers numerous benefits for overall health and well-being, including:

1. **Nutrient-Rich:** Plant-based diets are rich in essential nutrients such as vitamins, minerals, fiber, and antioxidants, supporting overall health and vitality.

2. **Heart Health:** Plant-based eating has been associated with a reduced risk of heart disease. The emphasis on fruits, vegetables, whole grains, and legumes helps lower cholesterol levels and supports cardiovascular health.

3. **Weight Management:** Many plant-based foods are low in calories and high in fiber, promoting satiety and making it easier to manage weight. Plant-based diets are often linked to maintaining a healthy weight.

4. **Digestive Health:** The fiber content in plant foods supports a healthy digestive system by promoting regular bowel movements and aiding in digestion.

5. **Reduced Inflammation:** Plant-based diets are often anti-inflammatory, helping to reduce inflammation in the body. Numerous health issues are associated with chronic inflammation.

6. **Blood Sugar Control:** Plant-based diets, particularly those rich in whole grains, fruits, and vegetables, can contribute to better blood sugar

control, making them beneficial for individuals with or at risk of diabetes.

7. **Disease Prevention:** Plant-based eating has been linked to a reduced risk of chronic diseases such as type 2 diabetes, certain cancers, and hypertension.

8. **Improved Energy Levels:** The nutrients obtained from plant-based foods contribute to sustained energy levels throughout the day, promoting overall vitality.

9. **Environmental Sustainability:** Plant-based diets typically have a lower environmental impact, as they require fewer natural resources and generate fewer greenhouse gas emissions compared to animal-based diets.

10. **Ethical Considerations:** Choosing plant-based options aligns with ethical considerations, promoting a more compassionate approach to food consumption and reducing the environmental impact of animal agriculture.

It's important to note that individual responses to diet can vary, and it's advisable to consult with a healthcare professional or a registered dietitian when making significant changes to your eating habits.

GETTING STARTED WITH PLANT-BASED COOKING

Embarking on a plant-based cooking journey is a rewarding endeavor. To get you going, consider the following guide:

1. **Educate Yourself:** Learn about the principles of plant-based eating. Understand the key food groups, essential nutrients, and how to create balanced meals without animal products.

2. **Stock Your Kitchen:** Ensure your kitchen is well-equipped with staples such as whole grains, legumes, a variety of fruits and vegetables, nuts, seeds, and plant-based proteins like tofu or tempeh.

3. **Experiment with Flavors:** Plant-based cooking opens up a world of diverse and delicious flavors. Experiment with herbs, spices, and condiments to enhance the taste of your dishes.

4. **Start Simple:** Begin with familiar recipes and gradually incorporate more plant-based ingredients. Simple dishes like stir-fries, salads, and grain bowls are great starting points.

5. **Explore Plant Proteins:** Discover a variety of plant-based protein sources such as beans, lentils, quinoa, and chickpeas. Experiment with different cooking methods to find your favorites.

6. **Plan Balanced Meals:** Ensure your meals include a mix of vegetables, fruits, whole grains, and protein sources to provide a well-rounded and satisfying dining experience.

7. **Meal Prep:** Consider batch cooking and meal prepping to make plant-based eating convenient during busy days. Having prepared ingredients can streamline the cooking process.

8. **Learn New Cooking Techniques:** Familiarize yourself with techniques like roasting, sautéing, and blending to create diverse textures and flavors in your plant-based dishes.

9. **Explore Plant-Based Alternatives:** Discover plant-based alternatives for dairy, such as almond or oat milk, and experiment with plant-based cheeses and meat substitutes if desired.

10. **Connect with the Community:** Join online forums or local groups to connect with others on a plant-based journey. Share experiences, recipes, and tips for a supportive community.

Recall that switching to a plant-based diet is a personal experience. Enjoy the process of exploring new flavors, nourishing your body, and discovering the diverse world of plant-based cuisine.

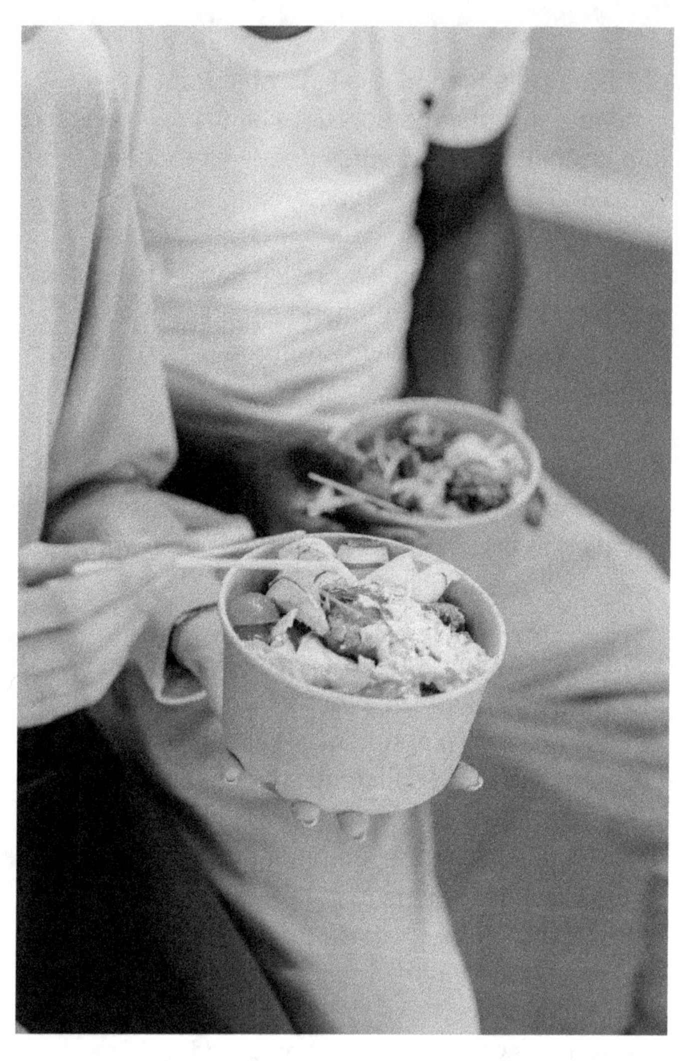

CHAPTER ONE

ESSENTIAL INGREDIENTS

Building a plant-based pantry is key to creating flavorful and nutritious meals. Here are essential ingredients to have on hand:

1. **Whole Grains:**
   - Brown rice
   - Quinoa
   - Whole wheat pasta
   - Barley
   - Oats

2. **Legumes:**
   - Lentils
   - Chickpeas
   - Black beans
   - Kidney beans
   - Cannellini beans

3. **Plant-Based Proteins:**
   - Tofu
   - Tempeh
   - Edamame
   - Plant-based protein powder (optional)

4. **Nuts and Seeds:**
   - Almonds
   - Walnuts

  - Chia seeds
  - Flaxseeds
  - Sunflower seeds

5. **Healthy Fats:**
   - Avocado
   - Olive oil
   - Coconut oil
   - Flaxseed oil

6. **Vegetables (Fresh and Frozen):**
   - leafy vegetables (collard, kale, and spinach)
   - Broccoli
   - Bell peppers
   - Carrots
   - Tomatoes

7. **Fruits (Fresh and Frozen):**
   - Berries
   - Apples
   - Bananas
   - Citrus fruits
   - Avocado

8. **Herbs and Spices:**
   - Garlic
   - Onion
   - Cumin
   - Turmeric
   - Paprika
   - Basil
   - Oregano

- Rosemary
- Thyme

9. **Plant-Based Milk Alternatives:**
   - Almond milk
   - Soy milk
   - Oat milk
   - Coconut milk

10. **Condiments and Sauces:**
    - Tamari or soy sauce
    - Balsamic vinegar
    - Nutritional yeast
    - Tahini
    - Mustard

11. **Whole Food Sweeteners:**
    - Maple syrup
    - Agave nectar
    - Dates

12. **Whole-Grain Flour:**
    - Whole wheat flour
    - Almond flour
    - Oat flour

13. **Plant-Based Dairy Alternatives:**
    - Plant-based yogurts
    - Non-dairy cheeses
    - Plant-based butter

14. **Canned Goods:**

  - Diced tomatoes
  - Tomato paste
  - Coconut milk
  - Vegetable broth

Having these essential ingredients readily available will empower you to create a wide range of delicious and nutritious plant-based meals. Adjust based on your preferences and explore new additions as you continue your plant-based cooking journey.

PROTEIN SOURCES

Getting an ample supply of protein is crucial in a plant-based diet. Here are diverse and nutritious plant-based protein sources:

1. **Legumes:**
   - Lentils
   - Chickpeas
   - Black beans
   - Kidney beans
   - Split peas

2. **Tofu:**
   - Firm, extra-firm, or silken tofu can be used in various dishes, absorbing the flavors of your recipes.

3. **Tempeh:**

   - A fermented soy product with a nutty flavor and firm texture, perfect for grilling, stir-frying, or crumbling into dishes.

4. **Edamame:**
   - Young, green soybeans packed with protein, often available frozen and great as a snack or in salads.

5. **Quinoa:**
   - A complete protein, containing all essential amino acids. Cook quinoa as a base for salads, bowls, or use it as a side dish.

6. **Seitan:**
   - Made from gluten, seitan has a meaty texture and is rich in protein. It's versatile and can be used in various savory dishes.

7. **Chia Seeds:**
   - Rich in omega-3 fatty acids and protein. Mix with liquid to create a gel-like consistency, ideal for puddings and smoothies.

8. **Hemp Seeds:**
   - Packed with protein, omega-3, and omega-6 fatty acids. Blend into smoothies or sprinkle over yogurt and salads.

9. **Black Rice:**

   - Also known as forbidden rice, black rice is higher in protein compared to other rice varieties and adds a unique color to dishes.

10. **Peanut Butter:**
   - A tasty spread that can add protein to your diet. Select natural peanut butter that doesn't have any additional sugars or oils.

11. **Almonds:**
   - Almonds are not only a healthy snack but also a good source of protein. Enjoy them on their own or as almond butter.

12. **Soy Milk:**
   - Fortified soy milk is a good plant-based milk alternative rich in protein. Use it in smoothies, coffee, or cereal.

13. **Green Peas:**
   - A versatile vegetable that can be added to salads, stir-fries, or enjoyed as a side dish.

14. **Plant-Based Protein Powder:**
   - A convenient option for adding extra protein to smoothies or recipes. Look for varieties made from pea, rice, or hemp protein.

By incorporating a variety of these plant-based protein sources into your meals, you can ensure you're meeting your protein needs while enjoying a diverse and delicious range of foods.

WHOLE GRAINS

Whole grains are a vital component of a plant-based diet, providing essential nutrients and dietary fiber. Here are some versatile and nutritious whole grains to include in your meals:

1. **Brown Rice:**
   - A staple with a nutty flavor, perfect as a side dish or as a base for bowls.

2. **Quinoa:**
   - a complete protein that has every necessary amino acid. Quick-cooking and versatile, suitable for salads, bowls, or as a side.

3. **Oats:**
   - A hearty grain packed with fiber, great for breakfast in the form of oatmeal, granola, or overnight oats.

4. **Barley:**
   - A chewy grain with a nutty flavor, ideal for soups, stews, and salads.

5. **Buckwheat:**
   - Despite the name, buckwheat is gluten-free. Use it in porridge, pancakes, or as a base for salads.

6. **Farro:**
   - A ancient wheat grain with a chewy texture, suitable for salads, soups, and pilafs.

7. **Freekeh:**
   - A roasted green wheat with a smoky flavor, excellent in salads or as a side dish.

8. **Millet:**
   - A small, versatile grain with a slightly sweet flavor. Cooked millet can be used in pilafs, salads, or as a breakfast porridge.

9. **Wild Rice:**
   - A nutrient-dense option with a robust, earthy flavor. Use it in pilafs or mix with other grains.

10. **Sorghum:**
    - A gluten-free grain with a mild taste, suitable for salads, bowls, or as a side dish.

11. **Spelt:**
    - An ancient wheat variety with a nutty flavor. Use spelt flour in baking or cook spelt berries for salads and sides.

12. **Amaranth:**
    - A tiny grain packed with protein and fiber. Cook amaranth as a porridge or use it in baking.

13. **Brown Bulgur:**

- Precooked and dried cracked wheat, ideal for quick and nutritious salads or side dishes.

14. **Teff:**
   - A small grain with a mildly nutty flavor, often used in Ethiopian cuisine. Cook teff as a side dish or use teff flour in baking.

Incorporating a variety of these whole grains into your meals ensures a diverse range of nutrients, textures, and flavors, contributing to a well-rounded and satisfying plant-based diet.

NUTRITIONAL POWERHOUSES: VEGETABLES AND FRUITS

Vegetables and fruits are nutritional powerhouses, brimming with vitamins, minerals, and antioxidants. Here are some vibrant options to elevate your plant-based meals:

Vegetables:

1. **Leafy Greens:**
   - Spinach
   - Kale
   - Swiss chard
   - Collard greens

2. **Cruciferous Vegetables:**
   - Broccoli
   - Cauliflower

- Brussels sprouts
- Cabbage

3. **Root Vegetables:**
   - Sweet potatoes
   - Carrots
   - Beets
   - Radishes

4. **Colorful Peppers:**
   - Bell peppers (red, yellow, green)
   - Chili peppers

5. **Tomatoes:**
   - Fresh tomatoes
   - Cherry tomatoes
   - Sun-dried tomatoes

6. **Onions and Garlic:**
   - Red onions
   - White onions
   - Garlic cloves

7. **Mushrooms:**
   - Portobello
   - Shiitake
   - Button mushrooms

8. **Zucchini and Squash:**
   - Zucchini
   - Yellow squash
   - Butternut squash

9. **Asparagus:**
   - A versatile green vegetable rich in nutrients.

10. **Avocado:**
   - Packed with healthy fats and a creamy texture, perfect for salads and spreads.

Fruits:

1. **Berries:**
   - Blueberries
   - Strawberries
   - Raspberries
   - Blackberries

2. **Citrus Fruits:**
   - Oranges
   - Grapefruits
   - Lemons
   - Limes

3. **Tropical Fruits:**
   - Pineapple
   - Mango
   - Papaya
   - Kiwi

4. **Apples and Pears:**
   - Enjoy these as snacks or incorporate them into salads and desserts.

5. **Bananas:**
   - A versatile fruit for smoothies, desserts, and snacking.

6. **Stone Fruits:**
   - Peaches
   - Plums
   - Nectarines
   - Apricots

7. **Grapes:**
   - Red or green, grapes are a sweet and refreshing addition to meals.

8. **Melons:**
   - Watermelon
   - Cantaloupe
   - Honeydew

9. **Pomegranate Seeds:**
   - Bursting with antioxidants, add these to salads or enjoy as a snack.

10. **Cherries:**
   - Sweet and tart, cherries are delightful on their own or in various dishes.

Incorporating a colorful array of vegetables and fruits ensures a diverse range of nutrients, flavors, and textures, making your plant-based meals not only nutritious but also delicious.

PLANT-BASED FATS

Plant-based fats are essential for a well-rounded and healthy plant-based diet. Here are some nutritious sources of plant-based fats:

1. **Avocado:**
   - Rich in monounsaturated fats, avocados add creaminess to dishes and provide a host of nutrients.

2. **Nuts:**
   - Almonds, walnuts, cashews, and pistachios offer healthy fats, protein, and various vitamins and minerals.

3. **Seeds:**
   - Chia seeds, flaxseeds, pumpkin seeds, and sunflower seeds are excellent sources of omega-3 fatty acids and other essential nutrients.

4. **Nut Butters:**
   - Peanut butter, almond butter, and other nut butters are versatile spreads rich in healthy fats.

5. **Olive Oil:**
   - Extra virgin olive oil is a staple in Mediterranean cuisine, providing monounsaturated fats and antioxidants.

6. **Coconut:**

   - Coconut oil, coconut milk, and shredded
coconut are rich in saturated fats but can be part of
a balanced plant-based diet in moderation.

7. **Flaxseed Oil:**
   - A plant-based oil high in omega-3 fatty acids,
often used as a supplement or added to smoothies.

8. **Chia Seeds:**
   - Besides being a great source of healthy fats,
chia seeds absorb liquid to form a gel-like
consistency, making them useful in puddings and
beverages.

9. **Hemp Seeds:**
   - Hemp seeds offer a balanced ratio of omega-3
and omega-6 fatty acids along with protein and
minerals.

10. **Dark Chocolate:**
   - Opt for dark chocolate with a high cocoa
content for a tasty source of plant-based fats and
antioxidants.

11. **Soybeans and Tofu:**
   - Whole soy products like edamame and tofu
contain healthy fats along with protein.

12. **Algal Oil:**
   - Derived from algae, algal oil is a plant-based
source of omega-3 fatty acids, suitable for
supplementation.

13. **Walnut Oil:**
   - Walnut oil is a flavorful option rich in omega-3 fatty acids, ideal for dressings and drizzling.

14. **Olives:**
   - Whether whole or as olive oil, olives provide monounsaturated fats and are a savory addition to many dishes.

Balancing these plant-based fats with other macronutrients ensures a well-rounded diet that supports overall health and provides sustained energy.

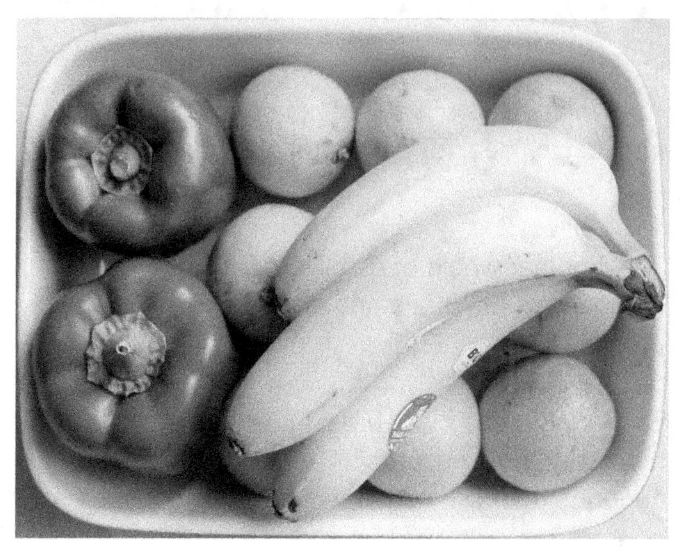

CHAPTER TWO

KITCHEN TOOLS AND TECHNIQUES

Creating delicious plant-based meals is made easier with the right kitchen tools and techniques. For your reference, consider this guide:

Kitchen Tools:

1. **High-Quality Blender:**
   - Ideal for smoothies, soups, sauces, and creamy plant-based desserts.

2. **Food Processor:**
   - Useful for chopping, shredding, and blending ingredients, especially nuts and vegetables.

3. **Chef's Knife:**
   - A sharp, versatile knife for chopping, dicing, and slicing vegetables and fruits.

4. **Cutting Boards:**
   - Have a selection of cutting boards for different ingredients to prevent cross-contamination.

5. **Vegetable Peeler:**
   - Handy for peeling vegetables or creating thin ribbons for salads.

6. **Quality Pots and Pans:**
   - Invest in a variety of sizes for cooking grains, simmering sauces, and sautéing vegetables.

7. **Steamer Basket:**
   - Preserves the nutrients in vegetables while cooking and is great for batch cooking.

8. **Baking Sheets:**
   - Essential for roasting vegetables, grains, and making plant-based desserts.

9. **Spatulas and Wooden Spoons:**
   - Perfect for stirring, flipping, and serving without scratching your cookware.

10. **Citrus Juicer:**
   - Extracts fresh juice for dressings, marinades, or beverages.

11. **Zester/Grater:**
   - Adds citrus zest or grates nuts for extra flavor and texture.

12. **Measuring Cups and Spoons:**
   - Precise measurements are crucial, especially in baking.

13. **Silicone Baking Mats:**
   - Non-stick and reusable for baking without added oils.

14. **Colander:**
   - Essential for draining pasta, rinsing grains, and washing fruits and vegetables.

Kitchen Techniques:

1. **Batch Cooking:**
   - Prepare ingredients in larger quantities to save time throughout the week.

2. **Meal Prepping:**
   - Portion out meals in advance for easy grab-and-go options.

3. **Sauteing:**
   - Use a small amount of oil or vegetable broth to cook vegetables quickly over medium heat.

4. **Roasting:**
   - Enhance flavors by roasting vegetables or even fruits in the oven.

5. **Blending and Pureeing:**
   - Create smooth sauces, soups, and dressings with a blender or food processor.

6. **Grilling:**
   - Achieve a smoky flavor by grilling vegetables, fruits, or plant-based proteins.

7. **Marinating:**

- Allow plant-based proteins to soak up flavors by marinating them before cooking.

8. **Sautéing:**
   - Quickly cook vegetables in a pan with a small amount of oil for a flavorful and nutritious side.

9. **Steaming:**
   - Preserve nutrients by steaming vegetables over boiling water.

10. **One-Pot Meals:**
   - Simplify cleanup by cooking everything in one pot or pan.

By combining the right tools with these essential techniques, you'll be well-equipped to create a wide variety of delicious and nutritious plant-based meals.

COOKING BASICS

Mastering cooking basics lays a solid foundation for creating delicious plant-based meals. Here are some fundamental cooking techniques to enhance your culinary skills:

1. **Knife Skills:**
   - Learn basic knife cuts like chopping, mincing, dicing, and julienning for efficient meal preparation.

2. **Sautéing:**
   - Cook ingredients quickly in a pan with a small amount of oil over medium heat, stirring frequently.

3. **Roasting:**
   - Use the oven to cook vegetables, grains, and even fruits by placing them on a baking sheet with a drizzle of oil.

4. **Steaming:**
   - Preserve nutrients by cooking vegetables over boiling water or using a steamer basket.

5. **Boiling and Simmering:**
   - Boil ingredients like pasta or grains in water, and simmer by reducing heat for longer, slower cooking.

6. **Blending and Pureeing:**
   - Use a blender or food processor to create smooth sauces, soups, or dressings.

7. **Grilling:**
   - Achieve a smoky flavor by cooking vegetables, fruits, or plant-based proteins on a grill or grill pan.

8. **Baking:**
   - Utilize the oven to bake grains, vegetables, and desserts like plant-based cookies or cakes.

9. **Marinating:**

- Enhance flavors by allowing plant-based proteins to soak in a mixture of herbs, spices, and liquids before cooking.

10. **Seasoning:**
   - Master the art of balancing flavors with herbs, spices, salt, and acid (lemon juice, vinegar) to elevate your dishes.

11. **Meal Prep:**
   - Plan and prepare ingredients in advance to streamline cooking during busy days.

12. **Sauteing:**
   - Quickly cook vegetables or tofu in a pan with a small amount of oil over medium heat for a flavorful side.

13. **Deglazing:**
   - Add liquid (such as broth or wine) to a hot pan to lift flavorful bits stuck to the bottom, creating a tasty sauce.

14. **Resting:**
   - Allow cooked plant-based proteins to rest before serving to retain juices and tenderness.

15. **Tasting and Adjusting:**
   - Taste your dishes as you cook and adjust seasonings to achieve the desired flavor.

Building confidence in these basic cooking techniques will empower you to create a wide range of plant-based dishes with ease. Experiment, embrace creativity, and enjoy the process of discovering your unique cooking style.

MUST HAVE KITCHEN EQUIPMENTS

Equip your kitchen with essential tools to streamline your plant-based cooking adventures. Here are must-have kitchen equipment:

1. **Chef's Knife:**
   - A high-quality, sharp knife for chopping, dicing, and slicing vegetables, fruits, and more.

2. **Cutting Boards:**
   - Have different cutting boards for vegetables, fruits, and other ingredients to prevent cross-contamination.

3. **Blender:**
   - Ideal for smoothies, sauces, soups, and creamy plant-based desserts.

4. **Food Processor:**
   - Great for chopping, shredding, and blending ingredients, especially nuts and vegetables.

5. **Pots and Pans:**

- A variety of sizes for boiling, simmering, sautéing, and other cooking methods.

6. **Baking Sheets and Pans:**
   - Essential for roasting vegetables, baking grains, and creating plant-based desserts.

7. **Silicone Baking Mats:**
   - Non-stick and reusable for baking without added oils.

8. **Steamer Basket:**
   - Preserves nutrients in vegetables while cooking and is great for batch cooking.

9. **Spatulas and Wooden Spoons:**
   - Essential for stirring, flipping, and serving without scratching your cookware.

10. **Measuring Cups and Spoons:**
   - For precise measurements in baking and cooking.

11. **Mixing Bowls:**
   - Multiple sizes for mixing ingredients, marinating, or preparing salads.

12. **Colander:**
   - Essential for draining pasta, rinsing grains, and washing fruits and vegetables.

13. **Strainer:**

- Useful for separating solids from liquids or straining sauces.

14. **Whisk:**
   - Incorporate air into mixtures, create smooth sauces, and blend ingredients.

15. **Tongs:**
   - Adaptable for serving, flipping, and rotating food.

16. **Peeler:**
   - Easily peel vegetables or create thin ribbons for salads.

17. **Citrus Juicer:**
   - Extract fresh juice for dressings, marinades, or beverages.

18. **Microplane Grater/Zester:**
   - Adds citrus zest or grates nuts for extra flavor and texture.

19. **Can Opener:**
   - A basic tool for opening canned ingredients.

20. **Digital Food Thermometer:**
   - Ensure proper cooking temperatures, especially for plant-based proteins.

21. **Vegetable Spiralizer:**

- Create noodles or ribbons from vegetables like zucchini or carrots.

Having these essential kitchen tools will make your plant-based cooking experience more efficient and enjoyable. As you explore different recipes, you may find additional tools that suit your cooking preferences and style.

FLAVORFUL SEASONINGS

Elevate your plant-based dishes with a variety of flavorful seasonings. Here are some essential seasonings to enhance the taste of your plant-based meals:

1. **Herbs:**
   - Basil
   - Thyme
   - Rosemary
   - Oregano
   - Parsley
   - Cilantro

2. **Spices:**
   - Cumin
   - Coriander
   - Paprika
   - Turmeric
   - Chili powder
   - Curry powder

3. **Garlic and Onion:**
   - Fresh garlic cloves
   - Garlic powder
   - Onion powder
   - Shallots

4. **Citrus:**
   - Lemon zest
   - Lime zest
   - Orange zest
   - Fresh lemon or lime juice

5. **Ginger:**
   - Fresh grated ginger
   - Ground ginger

6. **Chilies and Peppers:**
   - Red pepper flakes
   - Cayenne pepper
   - Jalapeños
   - Bell peppers

7. **Mustard:**
   - Dijon mustard
   - Whole grain mustard

8. **Vinegars:**
   - Balsamic vinegar
   - Apple cider vinegar
   - Red wine vinegar

9. **Soy Sauce and Tamari:**

- gives food more umami flavor and depth.

10. **Nutritional Yeast:**
   - Adds a cheesy flavor to plant-based dishes and is rich in B-vitamins.

11. **Cinnamon and Nutmeg:**
   - Perfect for adding warmth to desserts, oatmeal, or smoothies.

12. **Sesame Oil:**
   - Adds a rich, nutty flavor to stir-fries and Asian-inspired dishes.

13. **Herb Blends:**
   - Italian seasoning
   - Herbes de Provence
   - Garam masala

14. **Smoked Paprika:**
   - Infuses a smoky flavor to dishes without actual smoking.

15. **Tahini:**
   - A sesame seed paste that adds creaminess and nuttiness to sauces and dressings.

16. **Maple Syrup and Agave Nectar:**
   - Natural sweeteners that balance flavors in both sweet and savory dishes.

17. **Hot Sauce:**

- Enhances heat and flavor; choose your preferred level of spiciness.

18. **Tamari or Coconut Aminos:**
   - Provides a savory, umami taste similar to soy sauce.

19. **Capers and Olives:**
   - Add briny, salty flavors to Mediterranean-inspired dishes.

20. **Miso Paste:**
   - Creates a savory, umami-rich base for soups, stews, and marinades.

Experiment with these seasonings to create a symphony of flavors in your plant-based cooking. Adjust quantities based on your taste preferences and get creative with combinations to discover your signature dishes.

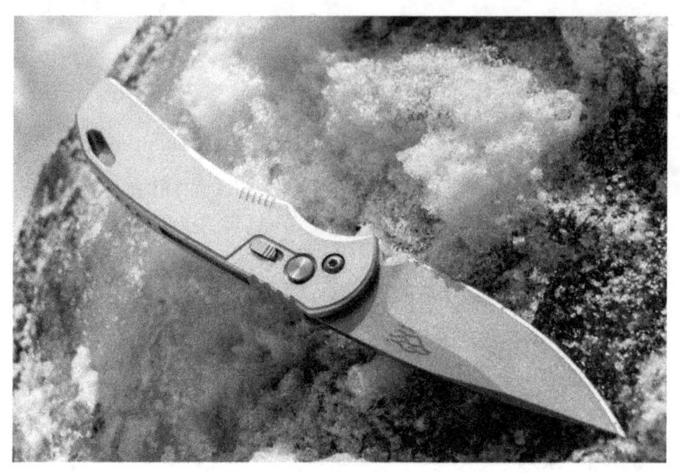

CHAPTER THREE

BREAKFAST FOR CHAMPIONS

Certainly! Here are five plant-based breakfast recipes with detailed instructions:

1. **Power-Packed Smoothie Bowl:**
  - ****Ingredients:****
    - 1 cup spinach
    - 1/2 cup kale
    - 1/2 cup frozen berries
    - 1 banana
    - 1 tablespoon chia seeds
    - 1 scoop plant-based protein powder
    - Granola, sliced almonds, almond butter (for topping)
  - ****Instructions:****
    1. Blend spinach, kale, berries, banana, chia seeds, and protein powder until smooth.
    2. Pour into a bowl and top with granola, sliced almonds, and a drizzle of almond butter.

2. **Avocado Toast Deluxe:**
  - ****Ingredients:****
    - 2 slices whole-grain bread
    - 1 ripe avocado
    - Cherry tomatoes
    - Radish slices
    - Nutritional yeast
    - Red pepper flakes

- Fresh fruit (for serving)
- **Instructions:**

1. Toast the bread slices.
2. Spread the avocado on the toast after mashing it.
3. Top with cherry tomatoes, radish slices, nutritional yeast, and red pepper flakes.
4. Serve with a side of fresh fruit.

3. **Protein-Packed Oatmeal:**
   - **Ingredients:**
     - 1 cup oats
     - Almond milk
     - Chia seeds, hemp seeds
     - Plant-based protein powder
     - Sliced bananas, berries
     - Almond butter
   - **Instructions:**

1. Cook oats with almond milk according to package instructions.
2. Stir in chia seeds, hemp seeds, and a scoop of protein powder.
3. Top with sliced bananas, berries, and a dollop of almond butter.

4. **Tofu Scramble Wrap:**
   - **Ingredients:**
     - Firm tofu
     - Turmeric, cumin, nutritional yeast
     - Whole-grain wrap
     - Spinach, tomatoes, avocado
   - **Instructions:**

1. Sauté crumbled tofu with turmeric, cumin, and nutritional yeast until golden.

2. Fill a wrap with tofu scramble, spinach, tomatoes, and avocado slices.

5. **Chia Pudding Parfait:**
  - ****Ingredients:****
    - Chia seeds
    - Almond milk
    - Coconut yogurt
    - Fresh fruit
    - Granola
  - ****Instructions:****

1. Mix chia seeds with almond milk and refrigerate overnight.

2. In the morning, layer chia pudding with coconut yogurt, fresh fruit, and granola.

Enjoy these energizing and nutritious breakfasts to start your day like a champion!

PROTEIN-PACKED SMOOTHIE BOWLS

Protein-Packed Smoothie Bowl

Ingredients:
- 1 cup spinach
- 1/2 cup kale
- 1 frozen banana

- Half a cup of frozen fruit, such strawberries or blueberries
- 1 tablespoon chia seeds
- 1 scoop plant-based protein powder
- One cup almond milk, or any other type of plant-based milk
- Toppings: Granola, sliced almonds, fresh berries, chia seeds, coconut flakes

Instructions:
1. **Blend the Smoothie Base:**
   - In a blender, combine spinach, kale, frozen banana, frozen berries, chia seeds, plant-based protein powder, and almond milk.
   - Blend until smooth and creamy. Adjust the consistency by, if necessary, adding extra almond milk.

2. **Prepare Toppings:**
   - While the smoothie is blending, gather your favorite toppings – granola, sliced almonds, fresh berries, chia seeds, and coconut flakes.

3. **Assemble the Bowl:**
   - Transfer the smoothie into a dish.
   - Arrange the toppings in an aesthetically pleasing manner, creating sections for each topping.

4. **Customize:**

- Get creative with your toppings. Add a drizzle of almond butter or a sprinkle of cinnamon for extra flavor.

5. **Enjoy:**
   - Grab a spoon and savor the protein-packed goodness of your smoothie bowl!

This protein-packed smoothie bowl is not only delicious but also provides a nutritious start to your day, keeping you energized and satisfied. Feel free to customize the recipe with your favorite fruits and toppings.

HEARTY OATMEAL VARIATIONS

Hearty Oatmeal Variations

Base Oatmeal Recipe:
- 1 cup rolled oats
- 2 cups almond milk (or any plant-based milk)
- Pinch of salt

Instructions:
1. **Cook Oats:**
   - In a saucepan, combine rolled oats, almond milk, and a pinch of salt.
   - Cook the oats over medium heat, stirring regularly, until they become creamy and the consistency you desire.

2. **Sweet and Nutty Oatmeal:**
   - Top your oatmeal with sliced bananas, chopped nuts (walnuts, almonds, or pecans), and a drizzle of maple syrup.

3. **Apple Cinnamon Oatmeal:**
   - Stir in diced apples while cooking the oats.
   - Top with a sprinkle of cinnamon, a handful of raisins, and a dollop of almond butter.

4. **Berry Bliss Oatmeal:**
   - Add a small amount of your preferred berry (strawberries, blueberries, or raspberries) to the mixture.
   - Top with a spoonful of coconut yogurt and a sprinkle of chia seeds.

5. **Pumpkin Spice Oatmeal:**
   - Add canned pumpkin puree and a dash of pumpkin spice to the oats.
   - Top with chopped pecans, a drizzle of maple syrup, and a sprinkle of cinnamon.

6. **Chocolate Banana Oatmeal:**
   - Stir in cocoa powder or chocolate protein powder to the oats.
   - Top with sliced bananas, a sprinkle of cacao nibs, and a drizzle of almond butter.

7. **Tropical Coconut Oatmeal:**
   - Mix in shredded coconut and a splash of coconut milk.

- Top with diced mango, pineapple chunks, and a sprinkle of macadamia nuts.

8. **Protein-Packed Peanut Butter Oatmeal:**
   - Swirl in a generous spoonful of peanut butter into the oats.
   - Top with sliced strawberries and a sprinkle of hemp seeds.

9. **Savory Spinach and Mushroom Oatmeal:**
   - Sauté mushrooms and spinach separately, then stir them into the cooked oats.
   - Season with salt, pepper, and a sprinkle of nutritional yeast.

10. **Citrus Burst Oatmeal:**
   - Stir in orange or grapefruit segments into the oats.
   - Top with a handful of pomegranate seeds and a drizzle of honey.

Serving Tip:
- Customize your oatmeal with additional toppings like sliced almonds, chia seeds, flaxseeds, or a splash of plant-based milk.

These hearty oatmeal variations offer a delightful range of flavors to keep your breakfasts interesting and satisfying. Adjust the ingredients to suit your taste preferences and enjoy a warm, nourishing bowl of oats to start your day.

Energizing Breakfast Burritos

Ingredients:
- Whole-grain tortillas
- One cup of washed, drained, and canned black beans
- one cup diced bell peppers (assorted colors)
- 1 cup diced tomatoes
- 1 cup spinach leaves
- 1 avocado, sliced
- 1 cup firm tofu, crumbled
- 1 tablespoon olive oil
- 1 teaspoon ground cumin
- 1 teaspoon smoked paprika
- Salt and pepper to taste
- Salsa and hot sauce for serving
- Fresh cilantro for garnish

Instructions:

1. **Prepare Tofu Scramble:**
   - In a skillet, heat olive oil over medium heat.
   - Add crumbled tofu and sauté until it starts to brown.
   - Season with ground cumin, smoked paprika, salt, and pepper.
   - Set aside.

2. **Sauté Vegetables:**

- If necessary, add a little extra olive oil to the same skillet.
   - Sauté diced bell peppers until they begin to soften.
   - Add spinach and cook until wilted.
   - Stir in black beans and diced tomatoes. Cook until heated through.

3. **Assemble Burritos:**
   - Warm the tortillas.
   - On each tortilla, layer the tofu scramble, sautéed vegetables, and sliced avocado.

4. **Fold and Roll:**
   - Fold the sides of the tortilla toward the center, then roll from the bottom to create a burrito.

5. **Serve:**
   - Serve the breakfast burritos with salsa, hot sauce, and a sprinkle of fresh cilantro.

6. **Enjoy:**
   - These energizing breakfast burritos are ready to be enjoyed, providing a satisfying mix of protein, fiber, and flavorful veggies to kickstart your day.

Feel free to customize your breakfast burritos with additional ingredients like vegan cheese, guacamole, or a squeeze of lime juice. These portable and nutritious burritos make for a convenient and delicious breakfast on the go.

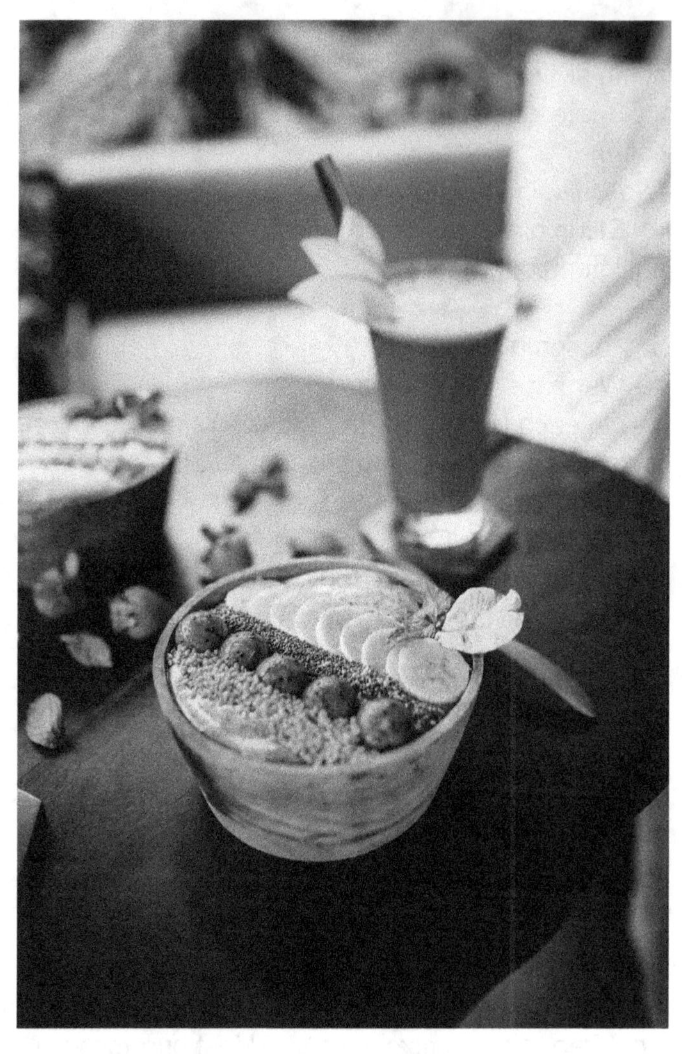

POWER-PACKED SMOOTHIES BOWLS

CHAPTER FOUR

POWER-PACKED LUNCHES

Certainly! Here are five power-packed plant-based lunch recipes with detailed instructions:

1. **Quinoa and Chickpea Salad Bowl:**
Ingredients:
- 1 cup cooked quinoa
- One cup of washed, drained, and canned chickpeas
- 1 cup cherry tomatoes, halved
- 1 cucumber, diced
- 1/2 red onion, finely chopped
- 1/4 cup Kalamata olives, sliced
- 1/4 cup fresh parsley, chopped
- Juice of 1 lemon
- 2 tablespoons extra-virgin olive oil
- Salt and pepper to taste
- Optional: Hummus for serving

Instructions:
1. In a large bowl, combine quinoa, chickpeas, cherry tomatoes, cucumber, red onion, olives, and parsley.
2. In a small bowl, whisk together lemon juice, olive oil, salt, and pepper.
3. Pour the dressing over the salad and toss until well combined.

4. Serve in bowls and drizzle with additional olive oil if desired. Optionally, add a dollop of hummus on top.

2. **Sweet Potato and Black Bean Buddha Bowl:**

Ingredients:
- 1 cup quinoa, cooked
- 1 large sweet potato, cubed
- One can of black beans, rinsed and drained
- 1 avocado, sliced
- 1 cup broccoli florets, steamed
- 1/4 cup pumpkin seeds
- Tahini dressing (3 tablespoons tahini, 1 tablespoon maple syrup, 2 tablespoons water)
- Salt and pepper to taste

Instructions:
1. Roast sweet potato cubes in the oven until tender.
2. Assemble bowls with quinoa, roasted sweet potato, black beans, avocado slices, steamed broccoli, and pumpkin seeds.
3. Drizzle with tahini dressing.
4. Season with salt and pepper, to taste.

3. **Mushroom and Spinach Stuffed Bell Peppers:**

Ingredients:
- Four big bell peppers, seeded and halved
- 2 cups quinoa, cooked
- 1 cup mushrooms, chopped

- 2 cups baby spinach, chopped
- One can of black beans, rinsed and drained
- 1 teaspoon cumin
- 1 teaspoon chili powder
- Salt and pepper to taste
- Salsa for topping

Instructions:
1. Preheat the oven to 375°F (190°C).
2. In a skillet, sauté mushrooms until they release moisture. Add spinach and cook until wilted.
3. In a bowl, mix cooked quinoa, sautéed mushrooms and spinach, black beans, cumin, chili powder, salt, and pepper.
4. Stuff bell peppers with the quinoa mixture.
5. Bake in the oven for 25-30 minutes or until peppers are tender.
6. Serve topped with salsa.

4. **Chickpea and Vegetable Stir-Fry:**
Ingredients:
- 2 cups cooked brown rice
- 1 can chickpeas, drained and rinsed
- 1 cup broccoli florets
- 1 bell pepper, sliced
- 1 carrot, julienned
- 1 cup snap peas, trimmed
- 2 tablespoons soy sauce
- 1 tablespoon sesame oil
- 1 teaspoon ginger, minced
- 2 cloves garlic, minced
- Green onions for garnish

Instructions:

1. Heat the sesame oil in a wok or big skillet over medium-high heat.

2. Add chickpeas, broccoli, bell pepper, carrot, snap peas, ginger, and garlic. Stir-fry until vegetables are tender-crisp.

3. Stir in cooked brown rice and soy sauce. Cook for an additional 2-3 minutes.

4. Before serving, sprinkle some chopped green onions on top.

5. **Lentil and Vegetable Curry:**

Ingredients:

- 1 cup dried lentils, rinsed
- 1 onion, chopped
- 2 bell peppers, diced
- 1 zucchini, diced
- 1 can coconut milk
- 1 can diced tomatoes
- 3 tablespoons curry powder
- 1 teaspoon turmeric
- 1 teaspoon cumin
- Salt and pepper to taste
- Fresh cilantro for garnish
- Brown rice or cooked quinoa to serve

Instructions:

1. In a large pot, sauté onions until softened.

2. Add bell peppers and zucchini, cooking until slightly tender.

3. Stir in curry powder, turmeric, and cumin until fragrant.
4. Add lentils, coconut milk, and diced tomatoes. Season with salt and pepper.
5. Simmer until lentils are cooked and vegetables are tender.
6. Serve over cooked quinoa or brown rice and garnish with fresh cilantro.

These power-packed lunch recipes provide a balance of nutrients and flavors to keep you energized throughout the day. Enjoy!

COLORFUL SALADS BOWLS

Colorful Rainbow Salad Bowl

Ingredients:
- **Base:**
  - Mixed salad greens (spinach, arugula, kale)
- **Vegetables:**
  - Cherry tomatoes, halved
  - Cucumber, sliced
  - Bell peppers (assorted colors), diced
  - Shredded purple cabbage
  - Carrot ribbons (use a peeler)
  - Radishes, thinly sliced
- **Proteins:**
  - Chickpeas, roasted
  - Quinoa, cooked
  - Edamame beans, steamed

- **Extras:**
  - Avocado, sliced
  - Fresh herbs (cilantro, mint, parsley)
  - Microgreens or sprouts
- **Dressing:**
  - Olive oil
  - Balsamic vinegar
  - Dijon mustard
  - Lemon juice
  - Salt and pepper to taste

Instructions:

1. **Prepare the Base:**
   - Arrange a generous handful of mixed salad greens as the base in each bowl.

2. **Add Vegetables:**
   - Place rows of cherry tomatoes, cucumber slices, diced bell peppers, shredded purple cabbage, carrot ribbons, and sliced radishes for a vibrant mix of colors.

3. **Include Proteins:**
   - Top the salad with roasted chickpeas, cooked quinoa, and steamed edamame beans for a protein boost.

4. **Layer on Extras:**
   - Arrange avocado slices, sprinkle fresh herbs, and add a handful of microgreens or sprouts for added texture and flavor.

5. **Prepare the Dressing:**
   - Whisk together olive oil, balsamic vinegar, Dijon mustard, lemon juice, salt, and pepper in a small bowl.

6. **Drizzle and Toss:**
   - Drizzle the dressing over each salad bowl just before serving.
   - To evenly coat all ingredients, lightly toss.

7. **Serve and Enjoy:**
   - Serve these colorful salad bowls immediately, celebrating the array of flavors and nutrients.

Feel free to customize the ingredients based on what's in season or your personal preferences. These rainbow salad bowls not only burst with color but also provide a variety of nutrients for a nourishing and visually appealing meal.

PROTEIN-RICH SANDWICHES AND WRAPS

Certainly! Here are two protein-rich sandwiches and wraps

Protein-Rich Chickpea Salad Wrap

Ingredients:

- 1 can (15 oz) chickpeas, drained and rinsed

- 1/4 cup vegan mayonnaise
- 1 tablespoon Dijon mustard
- 1 celery stalk, finely chopped
- 1/4 cup red onion, finely chopped
- 1 tablespoon fresh parsley, chopped
- Salt and pepper to taste
- Whole-grain wraps or tortillas
- Spinach or mixed greens
- Sliced tomatoes
- Avocado, sliced

Instructions:

1. **Prepare Chickpea Salad:**
   - Chickpeas should be mashed with a fork or potato masher in a bowl.
   - Add vegan mayonnaise, Dijon mustard, chopped celery, red onion, parsley, salt, and pepper. Mix well.

2. **Assemble Wraps:**
   - Lay out whole-grain wraps or tortillas.
   - Spread a generous amount of the chickpea salad onto each wrap.

3. **Add Greens and Veggies:**
   - Layer with spinach or mixed greens, sliced tomatoes, and avocado slices.

4. **Roll and Serve:**
   - Roll the wraps tightly, securing the fillings.
   - Slice in half and serve.

Enjoy these protein-packed chickpea salad wraps as a satisfying and wholesome lunch or dinner option.

Protein-Packed Grilled Tofu Sandwich

Ingredients:

- Firm tofu, sliced into 1/2-inch thick rectangles
- 2 tablespoons soy sauce
- 1 tablespoon olive oil
- 1 teaspoon smoked paprika
- 1/2 teaspoon garlic powder
- Whole-grain bread slices
- Vegan mayonnaise
- Mustard
- Lettuce leaves
- Sliced cucumbers
- Tomato slices
- Red onion, thinly sliced

Instructions:

1. **Marinate Tofu:**
   - In a bowl, whisk together soy sauce, olive oil, smoked paprika, and garlic powder.
   - Marinate tofu slices in the mixture for at least 15 minutes.

2. **Grill Tofu:**
   - Heat a skillet or grill pan over medium-high heat.

- Grill marinated tofu slices for about 3-4 minutes on each side, or until grill marks appear.

3. **Assemble Sandwiches:**
   - Spread vegan mayonnaise and mustard on whole-grain bread slices.
   - Layer grilled tofu, lettuce leaves, sliced cucumbers, tomato slices, and red onion.

4. **Serve and Enjoy:**
   - Slice the sandwiches in half and serve for a protein-rich and flavorful meal.

These protein-packed sandwich and wrap options are not only delicious but also provide a satisfying and nutrient-dense meal. Customize them with your favorite veggies and condiments for added variety.

HEARTY GRAIN BOWLS

Certainly! Here are two Hearty grain bowls recipes with detailed instructions

Hearty Mediterranean Quinoa Bowl

Ingredients:

- 1 cup cooked quinoa
- One cup of cooked or canned chickpeas (drained and rinsed)
- 1 cucumber, diced
- 1 cup cherry tomatoes, halved

- 1/2 cup Kalamata olives, sliced
- 1/4 cup red onion, finely chopped
- 1/4 cup fresh parsley, chopped
- 1/4 cup crumbled vegan feta cheese
- 2 tablespoons extra-virgin olive oil
- 1 tablespoon lemon juice
- 1 teaspoon dried oregano
- Salt and pepper to taste
- Hummus for serving

Instructions:

1. **Assemble Base:**
   - In a bowl, combine cooked quinoa, chickpeas, cucumber, cherry tomatoes, Kalamata olives, red onion, and fresh parsley.

2. **Prepare Dressing:**
   - Mix the olive oil, lemon juice, dried oregano, salt, and pepper in a small bowl.

3. **Drizzle and Toss:**
   - Pour the dressing into the combination of quinoa.
   -Gently toss to mix in all the ingredients.

4. **Top with Vegan Feta:**
   - Top with vegan feta cheese crumbles.

5. **Serve with Hummus:**
   - Serve the Mediterranean quinoa bowl with a side of hummus for extra flavor.

Hearty Buddha Bowl with Brown Rice

Ingredients:

- 1 cup cooked brown rice
- 1 cup baked sweet potato cubes
- 1 cup steamed broccoli florets
- 1/2 cup shredded carrots
- 1/2 cup edamame beans, shelled
- 1/4 cup sliced radishes
- 2 tablespoons tahini
- 1 tablespoon soy sauce
- 1 tablespoon rice vinegar
- 1 teaspoon maple syrup
- Sesame seeds for garnish

Instructions:

1. **Create Base:**
   - Arrange cooked brown rice as the base in a bowl.

2. **Add Vegetables:**
   - Top with baked sweet potato cubes, steamed broccoli, shredded carrots, edamame beans, and sliced radishes.

3. **Prepare Tahini Dressing:**
   - In a small bowl, whisk together tahini, soy sauce, rice vinegar, and maple syrup to create the dressing.

4. **Drizzle and Garnish:**
   - Over the bowl, drizzle the tahini dressing.
   - Garnish with sesame seeds.

5. **Enjoy:**
   - Toss the ingredients together before enjoying this wholesome Buddha bowl.

These hearty grain bowls are not only delicious but also packed with nutrients. Feel free to customize the ingredients based on your preferences and enjoy a nourishing and satisfying meal.

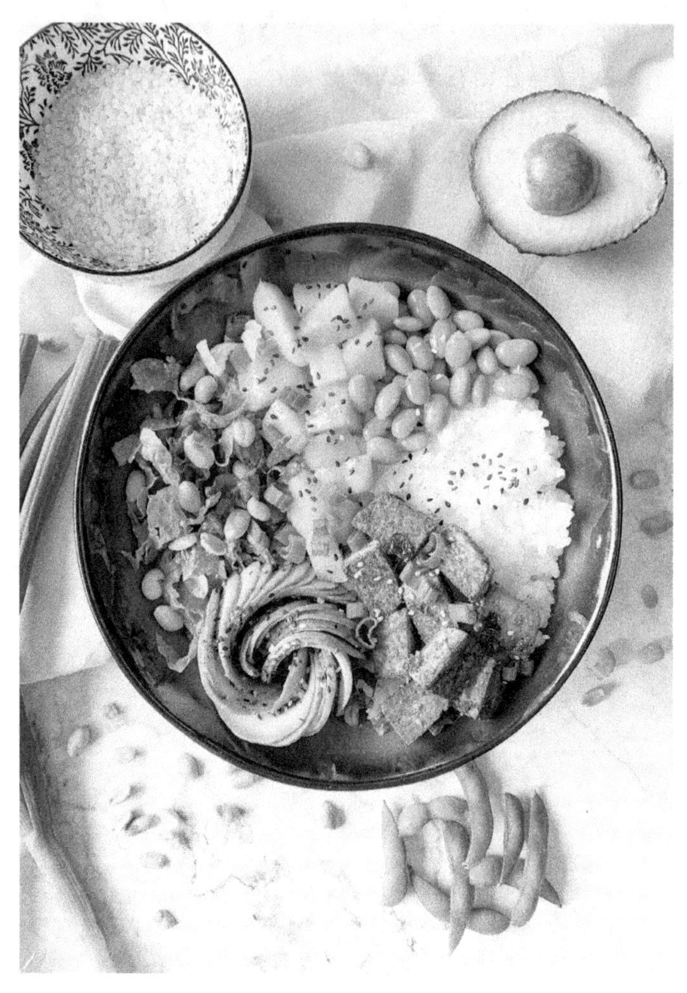

CHAPTER FIVE

MUSCLE-BUILDING DINNERS

Certainly! Here are four Muscle-building dinners recipes with detailed instructions.

1. **High-Protein Chickpea and Vegetable Stir-Fry**

ingredients:

- 1 can chickpeas, drained and rinsed
- 1 cup broccoli florets
- 1 bell pepper, sliced
- 1 carrot, julienned
- 1 cup snap peas, trimmed
- 2 tablespoons soy sauce
- 1 tablespoon olive oil
- 1 teaspoon ginger, minced
- 2 cloves garlic, minced
- Brown rice or quinoa for serving
- Sesame seeds for garnish

Instructions:

1. ****Stir-Fry Vegetables:****
   - In a wok or skillet, heat olive oil over medium-high heat.

   - Add chickpeas, broccoli, bell pepper, carrot, snap peas, ginger, and garlic. Stir-fry until vegetables are tender-crisp.

2. **Add Soy Sauce:**
   - Stir in soy sauce and continue cooking for an additional 2-3 minutes.

3. **Serve Over Grains:**
   - Serve the stir-fried vegetables and chickpeas over cooked brown rice or quinoa.

4. **Garnish:**
   - For some extra crunch and flavor, sprinkle sesame seeds on top.

2. **Grilled Lemon Herb Chicken with Sweet Potato Mash**

Ingredients:

- 4 boneless, skinless chicken breasts
- 2 lemons, juiced
- 2 tablespoons olive oil
- 2 teaspoons dried oregano
- 1 teaspoon dried thyme
- Salt and pepper to taste
- Quarter of a sweet potato, peeled and chopped
- 1/4 cup almond milk
- 2 tablespoons vegan butter

Instructions:

1. **Marinate Chicken:**
   - In a bowl, combine lemon juice, olive oil, dried oregano, dried thyme, salt, and pepper.
   - For a minimum of half an hour, marinate chicken breasts in the marinade.

2. **Grill Chicken:**
   - Grill chicken breasts until fully cooked, with grill marks on each side.

3. **Prepare Sweet Potato Mash:**
   - Steam or boil sweet potatoes until they become soft.
   - Mash sweet potatoes with almond milk and vegan butter.

4. **Serve:**
   - Serve grilled lemon herb chicken over a bed of sweet potato mash.

3. **Vegan Lentil and Vegetable Curry**

Ingredients:

- 1 cup dried green lentils, rinsed
- 1 onion, diced
- 2 bell peppers, diced
- 1 zucchini, diced
- 1 can coconut milk
- 1 can diced tomatoes

- 3 tablespoons curry powder
- 1 teaspoon turmeric
- 1 teaspoon cumin
- Salt and pepper to taste
- Fresh cilantro for garnish
- Brown rice for serving

Instructions:

1. **Sauté Vegetables:**
   - In a large pot, sauté diced onions until softened.
   - Add bell peppers and zucchini, cooking until slightly tender.

2. **Add Lentils and Spices:**
   - Stir in rinsed lentils, curry powder, turmeric, cumin, coconut milk, diced tomatoes, salt, and pepper.

3. **Simmer:**
   - Simmer until lentils are cooked and vegetables are tender.

4. **Serve Over Brown Rice:**
   - Over cooked brown rice, serve curry.

5. **Garnish:**
   - Garnish with fresh cilantro just before serving.

4. **Salmon and Quinoa Power Bowl**

Ingredients:

- 4 salmon fillets
- 1 cup quinoa, cooked
- 1 bunch asparagus, trimmed
- 1 tablespoon olive oil
- Lemon wedges for serving
- Salt and pepper to taste

Instructions:

1. **Grill Salmon and Asparagus:**
   - Use salt and pepper to season the salmon fillets.
   - Grill salmon and asparagus until cooked to your liking.

2. **Prepare Quinoa:**
   - To cook the quinoa, follow the instructions on the package.

3. **Assemble Power Bowl:**
   - Arrange cooked quinoa, grilled salmon, and asparagus in a bowl.

4. **Drizzle with Olive Oil:**
   - Drizzle with olive oil and squeeze lemon wedges over the top.

These muscle-building dinner options provide a good balance of protein, complex carbohydrates, and essential nutrients to support your fitness goals. Adapt serving quantities to your specific requirements and dietary choices.

PLANT-BASED PROTEIN MAIN COURSES

Certainly! Here are 4 Plant-Based protein main course recipes with instructions.

1. **Chickpea and Spinach Coconut Curry**

Ingredients:

- 1 can chickpeas, drained and rinsed
- 1 onion, finely chopped
- 2 cloves garlic, minced
- 1 tablespoon ginger, grated
- 1 can coconut milk
- 1 can diced tomatoes
- 2 cups baby spinach
- 2 teaspoons curry powder
- 1 teaspoon turmeric
- 1 teaspoon cumin
- Salt and pepper to taste
- Basmati rice for serving

Instructions:

1. **Sauté Aromatics:**
   - In a large pot, sauté chopped onion, garlic, and ginger until softened.

2. **Add Spices:**
   - Stir in curry powder, turmeric, cumin, salt, and pepper.

3. **Create Sauce:**
   - Add coconut milk and diced tomatoes (with their juice) to the pot.
   - Simmer for 10 minutes.

4. **Introduce Chickpeas and Spinach:**
   - Add chickpeas to the curry and cook until heated through.
   - Add baby spinach and stir until it wilts.

5. **Serve Over Basmati Rice:**
   - Arrange a bed of basmati rice for the curry.

2. **Lentil and Vegetable Stuffed Bell Peppers**

Ingredients:

- 4 bell peppers, cut in half, and seeds taken out
- One cup of rinsed and dry brown or green lentils
- 2 cups vegetable broth
- 1 onion, diced
- 2 cloves garlic, minced
- 1 zucchini, diced
- 1 carrot, grated
- 1 can diced tomatoes
- 1 teaspoon cumin
- 1 teaspoon smoked paprika

- Salt and pepper to taste
- Vegan cheese for topping (optional)

Instructions:

1. **Prepare Lentils:**
   - Cook lentils in vegetable broth until tender.

2. **Sauté Vegetables:**
   - In a skillet, sauté diced onion and minced garlic until softened.
   - Add diced zucchini and grated carrot, cooking until vegetables are tender.

3. **Combine Ingredients:**
   - Mix cooked lentils, sautéed vegetables, diced tomatoes, cumin, smoked paprika, salt, and pepper.

4. **Stuff Bell Peppers:**
   - Fill bell pepper halves with the lentil and vegetable mixture.

5. **Bake:**
   - Bake the peppers in the oven until they get soft.

6. **Optional: Add Vegan Cheese:**
   - If desired, sprinkle vegan cheese on top and bake until melted.

3. **Quinoa and Black Bean Stuffed Portobello Mushrooms**

Ingredients:

- 4 large portobello mushrooms, stems removed
- 1 cup quinoa, cooked
- One can of black beans, rinsed and drained
- 1 red bell pepper, diced
- One cup of corn kernels, either frozen or fresh
- 2 cloves garlic, minced
- 1 teaspoon cumin
- 1 teaspoon chili powder
- Salt and pepper to taste
- Avocado slices for topping
- Fresh cilantro for garnish

Instructions:

1. **Prepare Portobello Mushrooms:**
   - Preheat the oven and bake portobello mushrooms until tender.

2. **Cook Quinoa and Prepare Filling:**
   - To cook the quinoa, follow the instructions on the package.
   - In a skillet, sauté diced red bell pepper, corn, and minced garlic.
   - Add the cooked quinoa, black beans, chili powder, cumin, salt, and pepper.

3. **Stuff Mushrooms:**
   - Fill each portobello mushroom with the quinoa and black bean mixture.

4. **Bake:**
   - Bake until heated through.

5. **Top with Avocado and Garnish:**
   - Top with avocado slices and garnish with fresh cilantro.

4. **Tofu and Vegetable Stir-Fry with Brown Rice**

Ingredients:

- One block of cubed and pressed firm tofu
- 2 cups broccoli florets
- 1 bell pepper, sliced
- 1 carrot, julienned
- 1 cup snap peas, trimmed
- 2 tablespoons soy sauce
- 1 tablespoon sesame oil
- 1 teaspoon ginger, minced
- 2 cloves garlic, minced
- Brown rice for serving
- Sesame seeds for garnish

Instructions:

1. **Sauté Tofu:**
   - In a wok or skillet, sauté cubed tofu until golden.

2. **Stir-Fry Vegetables:**

- Add broccoli, bell pepper, carrot, snap peas, ginger, and garlic. Stir-fry until vegetables are tender-crisp.

3. **Add Soy Sauce and Sesame Oil:**
   - Drizzle with soy sauce and sesame oil. Toss to coat.

4. **Serve Over Brown Rice:**
   - Serve the tofu and vegetable stir-fry over cooked brown rice.

5. **Garnish:**
   - Sesame seeds can be used as a garnish to provide texture.

These plant based proteins provide a good balance of protein, complex carbohydrates, and essential nutrients to support your fitness goals. Adapt serving quantities to your specific requirements and dietary choices.

WHOLESOME GRAINS AND VEGETABLES COMBOS

Certainly! Here are 5 Wholesome Grains And Vegetables Combos

1. **Quinoa and Roasted Vegetable Bowl**

Ingredients:

- 1 cup quinoa, cooked
- 1 cup cherry tomatoes, halved
- 1 zucchini, sliced
- 1 red onion, diced
- 1 bell pepper, diced
- 2 tablespoons olive oil
- 1 teaspoon dried oregano
- Salt and pepper to taste
- Fresh basil for garnish

Instructions:

1. **Roast Vegetables:**
   - 200°C, or 400°F, should be the oven temperature.
   - Toss zucchini, red onion, and bell pepper with olive oil, dried oregano, salt, and pepper.
   - Roast in the oven for 20-25 minutes or until vegetables are caramelized.

2. **Assemble Bowl:**
   - Arrange cooked quinoa in bowls.
   - Add cherry tomatoes and roasted veggies on top.

3. **Garnish:**
   - Garnish with fresh basil before serving.

2. Brown Rice and Stir-Fried Tofu with Broccoli

Ingredients:

- 1 cup brown rice, cooked
- 1 block extra-firm tofu, cubed
- 2 cups broccoli florets
- 2 tablespoons soy sauce
- 1 tablespoon sesame oil
- 1 tablespoon rice vinegar
- 1 teaspoon ginger, minced
- 2 cloves garlic, minced
- Sesame seeds for garnish
- Green onions for garnish

Instructions:

1. **Stir-Fry Tofu and Broccoli:**
   - In a wok or skillet, stir-fry cubed tofu and broccoli with sesame oil until tofu is golden and broccoli is tender-crisp.

2. **Prepare Sauce:**
   - Combine soy sauce, rice vinegar, garlic, and ginger in a whisk.
   - Pour the sauce over the tofu and broccoli, tossing to coat.

3. **Serve Over Brown Rice:**
   - Serve the stir-fried tofu and broccoli over cooked brown rice.

4. **Garnish:**

- Before serving, garnish with green onions diced and sesame seeds.

3. **Couscous Salad with Mediterranean Vegetables**

Ingredients:

- 1 cup couscous, cooked
- 1 cucumber, diced
- 1 cup cherry tomatoes, halved
- 1 red bell pepper, diced
- 1/2 red onion, finely chopped
- 1/4 cup Kalamata olives, sliced
- 1/4 cup fresh parsley, chopped
- 2 tablespoons olive oil
- 1 tablespoon lemon juice
- Salt and pepper to taste
- Vegan feta cheese (optional)

Instructions:

1. **Prepare Couscous:**
   - Cook the couscous according to package directions.

2. **Combine Ingredients:**
   - In a large bowl, combine cooked couscous, cucumber, cherry tomatoes, red bell pepper, red onion, Kalamata olives, and fresh parsley.

3. **Make Dressing:**

   - To create the dressing, combine the olive oil, lemon juice, salt, and pepper in a mixing bowl.

4. **Toss and Chill:**
   - Pour the dressing over the couscous mixture and toss until well combined.
   - Refrigerate until it cools down before serving.

5. **Optional:**
   - If desired, crumble vegan feta cheese on top before serving.

4. **Wild Rice and Butternut Squash Pilaf**

Ingredients:

- 1 cup wild rice, cooked
- 1 small butternut squash, diced
- 1 red onion, diced
- 2 tablespoons olive oil
- 1 teaspoon dried thyme
- 1/2 teaspoon cinnamon
- Salt and pepper to taste
- Pomegranate seeds for garnish
- Chopped pecans for garnish

Instructions:

1. **Roast Butternut Squash:**
   - 200°C, or 400°F, should be the oven temperature.

- Toss diced butternut squash and red onion with olive oil, dried thyme, cinnamon, salt, and pepper.
   - Roast in the oven for 25-30 minutes or until squash is tender.

2. **Mix with Wild Rice:**
   - In a large bowl, combine cooked wild rice with the roasted butternut squash mixture.

3. **Garnish:**
   - Garnish with pomegranate seeds and chopped pecans before serving.

5. **Barley and Grilled Vegetable Bowl**

Ingredients:

- 1 cup barley, cooked
- 1 eggplant, sliced
- 1 zucchini, sliced
- 1 yellow squash, sliced
- 1 red bell pepper, sliced
- 2 tablespoons balsamic vinegar
- 3 tablespoons olive oil
- 1 teaspoon dried rosemary
- Salt and pepper to taste
- Fresh mint for garnish

Instructions:

1. **Grill Vegetables:**

- Preheat the grill. Grill eggplant, zucchini, yellow squash, and red bell pepper until charred and tender.

2. **Cook Barley:**
   - As directed on the packaging, prepare the barley.

3. **Prepare Dressing:**
   - Whisk together balsamic vinegar, olive oil, dried rosemary, salt, and pepper.

4. **Combine and Toss:**
   - In a large bowl, combine cooked barley with grilled vegetables.
   - Pour the dressing over the mixture and toss until well coated.

5. **Garnish:**
   - Just before serving, garnish with fresh mint.

These wholesome grain and vegetable combos offer a variety of flavors and textures, providing a nutritious and satisfying meal. Customize the recipes based on your preferences and enjoy the goodness of grains and vegetables.

COMFORTING ONE POT MEALS

Certainly! Here are 5 comforting one pot meals with detailed instructions

1. **Vegetarian Chickpea and Spinach Stew**

Ingredients:

- 1 can chickpeas, drained and rinsed
- 1 onion, diced
- 2 carrots, sliced
- 2 celery stalks, chopped
- 3 cloves garlic, minced
- 1 can (14 oz) diced tomatoes
- 4 cups vegetable broth
- 1 teaspoon cumin
- 1 teaspoon paprika
- 1/2 teaspoon turmeric
- Salt and pepper to taste
- 2 cups fresh spinach
- 1 lemon, juiced
- Fresh parsley for garnish

Instructions:

1. **Sauté Vegetables:**
   - Add the onions, carrots, celery, and garlic to a large pot and sauté until softened.

2. **Add Chickpeas and Spices:**
   - Stir in chickpeas, diced tomatoes, vegetable broth, cumin, paprika, turmeric, salt, and pepper.

3. **Simmer:**
   - Bring the stew to a boil, then reduce heat and let it simmer for 15-20 minutes.

4. **Add Spinach and Lemon Juice:**
   - Add fresh spinach and lemon juice to the stew.
   - Stir until the spinach wilts.

5. **Garnish and Serve:**
   - Before serving, sprinkle some fresh parsley on top.

2. **One-Pot Lentil and Vegetable Curry**

Ingredients:

- 1 cup dried green lentils, rinsed
- 1 onion, diced
- 1 bell pepper, diced
- 1 zucchini, diced
- 1 can coconut milk
- 1 can diced tomatoes
- 3 tablespoons curry powder
- 1 teaspoon cumin
- 1 teaspoon turmeric
- Salt and pepper to taste
- Fresh cilantro for garnish
- Cooked rice for serving

Instructions:

1. **Sauté Vegetables:**
   - In a large pot, sauté diced onions until softened.
   - Add diced bell pepper and zucchini, cooking until slightly tender.

2. **Add Lentils and Spices:**
   - Stir in rinsed lentils, curry powder, cumin, turmeric, coconut milk, diced tomatoes, salt, and pepper.

3. **Simmer:**
   - Simmer until lentils are cooked and vegetables are tender.

4. **Garnish:**
   - Before serving, add some fresh cilantro as a garnish.

5. **Serve Over Rice:**
   - Over cooked rice, serve the lentil and vegetable curry.

3. **Hearty Mushroom and Barley Stew**

Ingredients:

- 1 cup pearl barley, rinsed
- 1 onion, diced
- 2 carrots, sliced
- 2 celery stalks, chopped
- 3 cloves garlic, minced
- 8 oz mushrooms, sliced
- 4 cups vegetable broth
- 1 teaspoon thyme
- 1 teaspoon rosemary
- Salt and pepper to taste

- 1 can (14 oz) diced tomatoes
- Fresh parsley for garnish

Instructions:

1. **Sauté Vegetables:**
   - Add the onions, carrots, celery, and garlic to a large pot and sauté until softened.

2. **Add Mushrooms and Barley:**
   - Add sliced mushrooms and rinsed pearl barley to the pot.

3. **Pour Broth and Add Spices:**
   - Pour vegetable broth into the pot.
   - Stir in the rosemary, salt, and pepper.

4. **Simmer:**
   - Simmer until barley is cooked and vegetables are tender.

5. **Stir in Tomatoes:**
   - Stir in diced tomatoes and heat through.

6. **Garnish and Serve:**
   - Before serving, sprinkle some fresh parsley on top.

4. **Vegan One-Pot Pasta Primavera**

Ingredients:

- 8 oz whole wheat pasta
- 1 onion, thinly sliced
- 1 bell pepper, thinly sliced
- 1 zucchini, julienned
- 1 carrot, julienned
- 2 cloves garlic, minced
- 4 cups vegetable broth
- 1 can (14 oz) diced tomatoes
- 1 teaspoon Italian seasoning
- Salt and pepper to taste
- Fresh basil for garnish

Instructions:

1. **Combine Ingredients:**
   - In a large pot, combine pasta, sliced onions, bell pepper, julienned zucchini, julienned carrot, minced garlic, vegetable broth, diced tomatoes, Italian seasoning, salt, and pepper.

2. **Bring to a Boil:**
   - After bringing the mixture to a boil, lower the heat and simmer it.

3. **Cook Until Pasta is Tender:**
   - Simmer until the vegetables are soft and the pasta is cooked.

4. **Garnish and Serve:**
   - Garnish with fresh basil before serving.

5. **Spicy Chickpea and Rice Skillet**

Ingredients:

- 1 cup basmati rice, uncooked
- 1 can chickpeas, drained and rinsed
- 1 onion, diced
- 1 bell pepper, diced
- 2 cloves garlic, minced
- 1 tablespoon olive oil
- 1 teaspoon cumin
- 1 teaspoon smoked paprika
- 1/2 teaspoon cayenne pepper
- 2 cups vegetable broth
- Salt and pepper to taste
- Fresh cilantro for garnish

Instructions:

1. **Sauté Vegetables:**
   - In a large skillet, sauté onions, bell pepper, and garlic in olive oil until softened.

2. **Add Chickpeas and Spices:**
   - Stir in chickpeas, cumin, smoked paprika, and cayenne pepper.

3. **Add Rice and Broth:**
   - Add basmati rice to the skillet and pour in vegetable broth.

4. **Simmer:**

  - Cook the rice and allow the liquid to be
absorbed by simmering it.

5. **Garnish and Serve:**
  - Before serving, add some fresh cilantro as a
garnish.

These comforting one-pot meals are not only easy
to prepare but also packed with wholesome
ingredients for a satisfying and nutritious dining
experience. Enjoy the convenience of simple
cooking without compromising on flavor!

CHAPTER SIX

SNACK ATTACK

Certainly! Here are 6 snacks recipes with instructions.

1. **Crispy Roasted Chickpeas**

Ingredients:

- 1 can chickpeas, drained and rinsed
- 1 tablespoon olive oil
- 1 teaspoon smoked paprika
- 1/2 teaspoon cumin
- 1/2 teaspoon garlic powder
- Salt to taste

Instructions:

1. **Preheat Oven:**
   - 200°C, or 400°F, should be the oven temperature.

2. **Dry and Season Chickpeas:**
   - Using a paper towel, pat the chickpeas dry.
   - In a bowl, toss chickpeas with olive oil, smoked paprika, cumin, garlic powder, and salt.

3. **Roast:**

   - Spread the seasoned chickpeas on a baking
sheet.
   - Roast in the oven for 25-30 minutes or until
crispy, shaking the pan halfway through.

4. **Cool and Enjoy:**
   - Allow the roasted chickpeas to cool before
enjoying this crunchy and protein-packed snack.

2. **Homemade Trail Mix

Ingredients:

- 1 cup almonds
- 1 cup walnuts
- 1/2 cup pumpkin seeds
- 1/2 cup dried cranberries
- 1/2 cup dark chocolate chips
- 1/2 teaspoon sea salt

Instructions:

1. **Mix Ingredients:**
   - In a bowl, combine almonds, walnuts, pumpkin
seeds, dried cranberries, and dark chocolate chips.

2. **Sprinkle Salt:**
   - Sprinkle sea salt over the mix and toss to
combine.

3. **Portion and Store:**
   - Portion the trail mix into snack-sized servings.

- For an easy and wholesome snack, store in an airtight container.

3. **Apple Slices with Almond Butter**

Ingredients:

- 2 apples, cored and sliced
- 1/4 cup almond butter

Instructions:

1. **Slice Apples:**
   - Core and slice the apples into wedges.

2. **Serve with Almond Butter:**
   - Dip apple slices into almond butter for a delicious and satisfying combination.

4. **Greek Yogurt Parfait**

Ingredients:

- 1 cup Greek yogurt
- 1/2 cup granola
- 1/2 cup mixed berries
- Honey for drizzling

Instructions:

1. **Layer Ingredients:**

  - In a glass or bowl, layer Greek yogurt, granola, and mixed berries.

2. **Drizzle with Honey:**
  - Pour some honey on top to provide a little sweetness.

3. **Enjoy:**
  - Enjoy this protein-rich and flavorful parfait as a snack.

5. **Vegetable Sticks with Hummus**

Ingredients:

- Carrot sticks
- Cucumber slices
- Bell pepper strips
- Cherry tomatoes
- Hummus for dipping

Instructions:

1. **Prepare Vegetables:**
  - Cut carrots, cucumber, and bell pepper into sticks or slices.
  - Leave cherry tomatoes whole.

2. **Serve with Hummus:**
  - Place the carrot sticks in a platter.
  - Serve with a side of hummus for a crunchy and satisfying snack.

6. **Baked Sweet Potato Chips**

Ingredients:

- 2 sweet potatoes, thinly sliced
- 2 tablespoons olive oil
- 1 teaspoon paprika
- 1/2 teaspoon sea salt

Instructions:

1. **Preheat Oven:**
   - 200°C, or 400°F, should be the oven temperature.

2. **Toss with Seasonings:**
   - In a bowl, toss sweet potato slices with olive oil, paprika, and sea salt.

3. **Bake:**
   - Arrange the seasoned sweet potato slices on a baking sheet.
   - Bake for 20-25 minutes or until the chips are crispy.

4. **Cool and Crunch:**
   - Allow the sweet potato chips to cool before indulging in this flavorful and guilt-free snack.

These snack ideas cover a range of flavors and textures, from crunchy roasted chickpeas to sweet

and satisfying apple slices with almond butter.
Choose the one that fits your cravings and enjoy a
delightful snack attack!

NUT AND SEED MIXES

Certainly! Here are 5 Nut and Seeds mixes recipes
with instructions.

1. **Classic Nut Mix**

Ingredients:

- 1 cup almonds
- 1 cup walnuts
- 1 cup cashews
- 1 cup pecans
- 1/2 teaspoon sea salt

Instructions:

1. **Combine Nuts:**
   - In a bowl, combine almonds, walnuts, cashews,
and pecans.

2. **Sprinkle Salt:**
   - Sprinkle sea salt over the nut mix and toss to
coat.

3. **Roast or Enjoy Raw:**

- Optionally, roast the mix in the oven at 350°F (175°C) for 10-12 minutes for added flavor, or enjoy it raw.

2. **Tropical Trail Mix**

Ingredients:

- 1 cup mixed nuts (almonds, cashews, macadamias)
- 1/2 cup dried pineapple, diced
- 1/2 cup dried mango, diced
- 1/2 cup coconut flakes
- 1/4 cup dark chocolate chips

Instructions:

1. **Combine Ingredients:**
   - In a bowl, combine mixed nuts, dried pineapple, dried mango, coconut flakes, and dark chocolate chips.

2. **Mix Well:**
   - Mixing the components well is necessary.

3. **Portion and Enjoy:**
   - Portion the tropical trail mix into snack-sized servings and enjoy this sweet and savory mix.

3. **Superseed Crunch Mix**

Ingredients:

- 1/2 cup pumpkin seeds (pepitas)
- 1/2 cup sunflower seeds
- 1/4 cup chia seeds
- 1/4 cup flaxseeds
- 1/4 cup sesame seeds
- 1 tablespoon maple syrup
- 1/2 teaspoon cinnamon
- Pinch of sea salt

Instructions:

1. **Mix Seeds:**
   - In a bowl, mix pumpkin seeds, sunflower seeds, chia seeds, flaxseeds, and sesame seeds.

2. **Add Sweetness and Spice:**
   - Drizzle maple syrup over the seeds and sprinkle with cinnamon and a pinch of sea salt.
   - Toss to coat evenly.

3. **Bake or Enjoy Raw:**
   - Optionally, bake the mix in the oven at 325°F (163°C) for 15-20 minutes, stirring halfway through, or enjoy it raw.

4. **Antioxidant Berry and Nut Mix**

Ingredients:

- One cup of mixed nuts (pistachios, walnuts, and almonds)

- 1/2 cup dried blueberries
- 1/2 cup dried cranberries
- 1/4 cup goji berries
- 1/4 cup dark chocolate-covered almonds

Instructions:

1. **Combine Ingredients:**
   - In a bowl, combine mixed nuts, dried blueberries, dried cranberries, goji berries, and dark chocolate-covered almonds.

2. **Mix Well:**
   - Mixing the components well is necessary.

3. **Portion and Enjoy:**
   - Portion the antioxidant berry and nut mix into snack-sized servings and savor the delicious blend of flavors.

5. **Spicy Cajun Seed Mix**

Ingredients:

- 1/2 cup pumpkin seeds (pepitas)
- 1/2 cup sunflower seeds
- 1/2 cup almonds
- 1 tablespoon olive oil
- 1 teaspoon Cajun seasoning
- 1/2 teaspoon smoked paprika
- 1/4 teaspoon cayenne pepper
- 1/4 teaspoon garlic powder

- Pinch of sea salt

Instructions:

1. **Coat Seeds and Nuts:**
   - In a bowl, coat pumpkin seeds, sunflower seeds, and almonds with olive oil.

2. **Add Spices:**
   - Sprinkle Cajun seasoning, smoked paprika, cayenne pepper, garlic powder, and a pinch of sea salt over the seeds and nuts. Toss to coat evenly.

3. **Roast or Enjoy Raw:**
   - Optionally, roast the mix in the oven at 325°F (163°C) for 12-15 minutes or until golden, stirring halfway through, or enjoy it raw.

These nut and seed mixes offer a variety of flavors and textures, from classic to tropical and spicy Cajun. They make for convenient, nutrient-packed snacks that are easy to prepare and enjoy on the go.

GUILT-FREE CHIPS AND DIPS

Certainly! Here are 5 Guilt-free chips and dips recipes with instructions.

1. Baked Kale Chips

Ingredients:

- One bundle of chopped and separated kale leaves
- 1 tablespoon olive oil
- 1/2 teaspoon sea salt
- 1/4 teaspoon garlic powder

Instructions:

1. **Preheat Oven:**
   - Preheat the oven to 350°F (175°C).

2. **Massage with Oil:**
   - In a bowl, massage kale pieces with olive oil until well coated.

3. **Season:**
   - Sprinkle sea salt and garlic powder over the kale and toss to coat.

4. **Bake:**
   - Spread the kale on a baking sheet and bake for 10-15 minutes or until crispy.

5. **Cool and Crunch:**
   - Allow the baked kale chips to cool before enjoying this guilt-free and crunchy snack.

2. **Sweet Potato Chips**

Ingredients:

- 2 medium sweet potatoes, thinly sliced
- 2 tablespoons olive oil
- 1/2 teaspoon paprika
- 1/2 teaspoon garlic powder
- 1/4 teaspoon sea salt

Instructions:

1. **Preheat Oven:**
   - Preheat the oven to 375°F (190°C).

2. **Coat with Oil and Season:**
   - In a bowl, coat sweet potato slices with olive oil.
   - Sprinkle paprika, garlic powder, and sea salt
over the slices. Toss to coat.

3. **Bake:**
   - Arrange the seasoned sweet potato slices on a
baking sheet.
   - Bake the chips for 15 to 20 minutes, or until they
become crispy.

4. **Cool and Enjoy:**
   - Allow the sweet potato chips to cool before
indulging in this flavorful and guilt-free snack.

3. **Cucumber Chips with Tzatziki Dip**

Ingredients:

- 2 large cucumbers, thinly sliced

- 1 cup Greek yogurt
- 1/2 cucumber, finely diced
- 2 tablespoons fresh dill, chopped
- 1 clove garlic, minced
- 1 tablespoon lemon juice
- Salt and pepper to taste

Instructions:

1. **Prepare Cucumbers:**
   - Slice the cucumbers thinly using a mandolin or knife.

2. **Make Tzatziki Dip:**
   - In a bowl, combine Greek yogurt, diced cucumber, chopped dill, minced garlic, lemon juice, salt, and pepper to create the tzatziki dip.

3. **Dip and Enjoy:**
   - Dip the cucumber chips into the tzatziki sauce for a refreshing and guilt-free snack.

4. **Roasted Chickpea Dip**

Ingredients:

- 1 can chickpeas, drained and rinsed
- 2 tablespoons olive oil
- 1 teaspoon cumin
- 1/2 teaspoon smoked paprika
- 1/4 teaspoon cayenne pepper
- Salt and pepper to taste

- 2 tablespoons tahini
- 1 clove garlic, minced
- 2 tablespoons lemon juice
- Water (as needed for consistency)

Instructions:

1. **Roast Chickpeas:**
   - First, preheat the oven to 400°F, or 200°C.
   - Toss chickpeas with olive oil, cumin, smoked paprika, cayenne pepper, salt, and pepper.
   - Roast in the oven for 25-30 minutes or until crispy.

2. **Make Chickpea Dip:**
   - In a food processor, blend roasted chickpeas, tahini, minced garlic, and lemon juice.
   - Add water as needed for a smooth and creamy consistency.

3. **Serve and Dip:**
   - Serve the roasted chickpea dip with veggie sticks or baked chips for a guilt-free and flavorful snack.

5. **Zucchini Chips with Guacamole**

Ingredients:

- 2 large zucchinis, thinly sliced
- 2 tablespoons olive oil
- 1/2 teaspoon garlic powder

- 1/2 teaspoon onion powder
- 1/4 teaspoon cayenne pepper
- Salt and pepper to taste
- 2 ripe avocados
- 1 clove garlic, minced
- 1 tablespoon lime juice
- 1/4 cup red onion, finely chopped
- 1/4 cup cilantro, chopped
- Salt and pepper to taste

Instructions:

1. **Prepare Zucchini Chips:**
   - Slice the zucchinis thinly using a mandolin or knife.

2. **Coat and Season Zucchini:**
   - In a bowl, coat zucchini slices with olive oil.
   - Sprinkle garlic powder, onion powder, cayenne pepper, salt, and pepper over the slices. Toss to coat.

3. **Bake:**
   - The seasoned zucchini slices should be arranged on a baking pan.
   - Bake the chips for 15 to 20 minutes, or until they become crispy.

4. **Make Guacamole:**
   - Peel and mash the avocados in a bowl.

  - Add minced garlic, lime juice, chopped red
onion, cilantro, salt, and pepper to create
guacamole.

5. **Dip and Enjoy:**
  - Dip the zucchini chips into the guacamole for a
satisfying and guilt-free snack.

These guilt-free chips and dips provide a tasty
alternative to traditional snacks, offering a satisfying
crunch with wholesome ingredients. Enjoy these
flavorful combinations without compromising on
health!

CREATIVE PLANT-BASED SNACK IDEAS

Certainly! Here are 5 creative plant-based snack
ideas recipes with instructions.

1. **Avocado and Tomato Bruschetta**

Ingredients:

- Baguette slices (whole grain or gluten-free)
- 2 ripe avocados, mashed
- Cherry tomatoes, sliced
- Fresh basil leaves, chopped
- Balsamic glaze for drizzling
- Salt and pepper to taste

Instructions:

1. **Toast Baguette Slices:**
   - Toast baguette slices until crispy.

2. **Spread Avocado:**
   - Spread mashed avocado on each toast.

3. **Top with Tomatoes and Basil:**
   - Place sliced cherry tomatoes and chopped fresh basil on top.

4. **Drizzle Balsamic Glaze:**
   - Drizzle with balsamic glaze and season with salt and pepper.

5. **Enjoy:**
   - Enjoy this flavorful and creative plant-based bruschetta snack.

2. **Stuffed Mini Bell Peppers**

Ingredients:

- Mini bell peppers
- Hummus
- Cherry tomatoes, halved
- Cucumber, diced
- Fresh parsley, chopped

Instructions:

1. **Prepare Bell Peppers:**

   - Remove the seeds after halving the small bell peppers.

2. **Fill with Hummus:**
   - Fill each side of a pepper with hummus.

3. **Top with Tomatoes and Cucumber:**
   - Place a halved cherry tomato and diced cucumber on top.

4. **Garnish:**
   - Garnish with chopped fresh parsley.

5. **Serve:**
   - Serve these colorful stuffed mini peppers as a delightful and nutritious snack.

3. **Spicy Roasted Chickpea Poppers**

Ingredients:

- Chickpeas, cooked or canned
- Olive oil
- Smoked paprika
- Cumin
- Cayenne pepper
- Garlic powder
- Salt and pepper

Instructions:

1. **Coat Chickpeas:**

   - Toss chickpeas with olive oil, smoked paprika, cumin, cayenne pepper, garlic powder, salt, and pepper.

2. **Roast:**
   - Bake the chickpeas until they get crispy.

3. **Spicy Pop:**
   - Enjoy these spicy roasted chickpea poppers for a protein-packed and flavorful snack.

4. **Crispy Baked Zucchini Fries**

Ingredients:

- Zucchini, cut into fries
- Almond flour
- Nutritional yeast
- Garlic powder
- Onion powder
- Paprika
- Salt and pepper

Instructions:

1. **Coat Zucchini:**
   - Coat zucchini fries with a mixture of almond flour, nutritional yeast, garlic powder, onion powder, paprika, salt, and pepper.

2. **Bake:**
   - Bake in the oven until crispy.

3. **Dip and Enjoy:**
   - Serve these crispy baked zucchini fries with your favorite plant-based dipping sauce.

5. **Fruit Sushi Rolls**

Ingredients:

- Nori sheets
- Cooked quinoa
- Mango slices
- Avocado slices
- Cucumber strips
- Sesame seeds

Instructions:

1. **Prepare Nori Sheets:**
   - Arrange a nori sheet onto a sushi roller made of bamboo.

2. **Add Quinoa and Fillings:**
   - Spread cooked quinoa on the nori sheet.
   - Add mango slices, avocado slices, and cucumber strips.

3. **Roll and Slice:**
   - Roll the nori sheet and slice into bite-sized fruit sushi rolls.

4. **Sprinkle Sesame Seeds:**

  - For extra crunch, sprinkle sesame seeds over the top.

5. **Soy Sauce Dip:**
  - Serve with a side of soy sauce for a unique and creative plant-based snack.

These creative plant-based snack ideas offer a variety of flavors and textures, making them both satisfying and enjoyable. Whether you're in the mood for savory or sweet, these snacks have you covered!

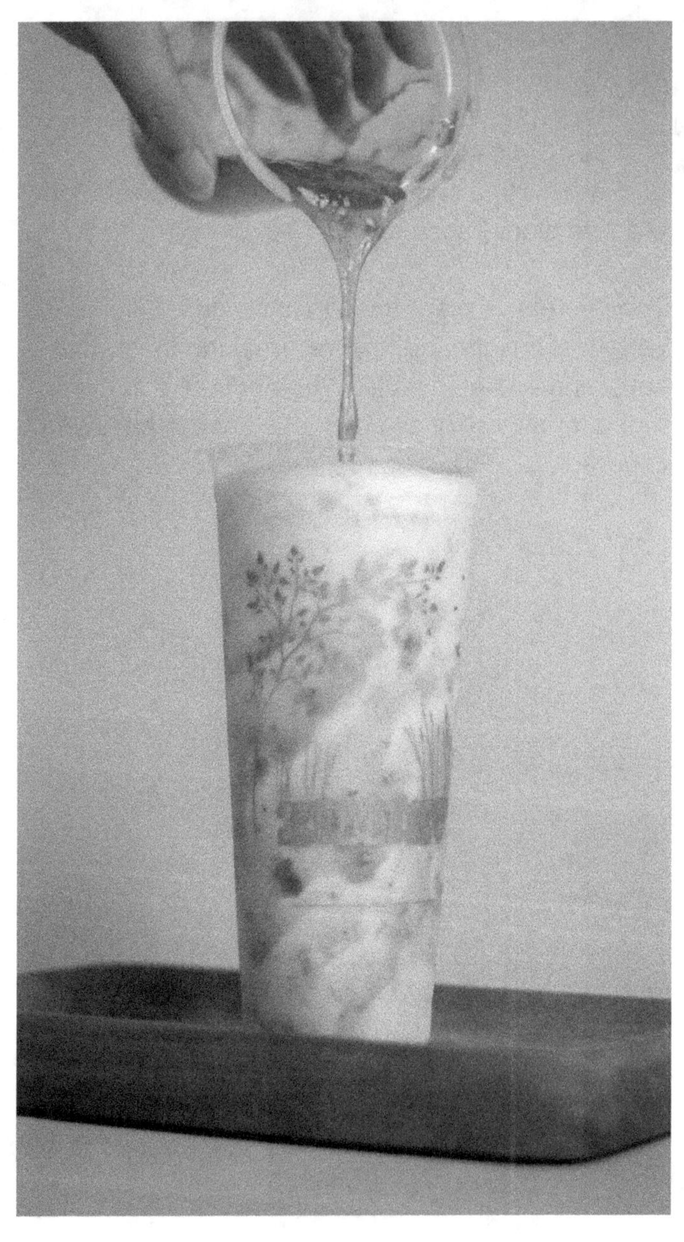

CHAPTER SEVEN

DESSERTS WITH A TWIST

Certainly! Here are 5 desserts recipes with instructions.

1. **Vegan Avocado Chocolate Mousse**

Ingredients:

- 2 ripe avocados
- 1/2 cup cocoa powder
- 1/4 cup maple syrup
- 1 teaspoon vanilla extract
- Pinch of salt
- Coconut whipped cream for topping (optional)

Instructions:

1. **Blend Ingredients:**
   - In a blender, combine avocados, cocoa powder, maple syrup, vanilla extract, and a pinch of salt.
   - Blend until smooth and creamy.

2. **Chill:**
   - Chill the chocolate mousse in the refrigerator for at least 1 hour.

3. **Serve:**

- Serve topped with coconut whipped cream for a rich and indulgent twist on chocolate mousse.

2. **Aquafaba Meringue Cookies**

Ingredients:

- Half a cup aquafaba, or chickpea can liquid
- 1/2 cup granulated sugar
- 1 teaspoon vanilla extract
- Vegan chocolate chips or chopped nuts (optional)

Instructions:

1. **Whip Aquafaba:**
   - Whip the aquafaba with a mixer until firm peaks form.

2. **Add Sugar and Flavor:**
   - Gradually add sugar while continuing to whip.
   - Add vanilla extract and mix until glossy.

3. **Pipe or Spoon:**
   - Pipe or spoon dollops onto a baking sheet.

4. **Bake:**
   - Bake in a preheated oven at 200°F (93°C) for 1.5 to 2 hours until the meringues are crispy.

5. **Cool and Enjoy:**

- Allow the meringues to cool and optionally dip in vegan chocolate or sprinkle with chopped nuts for a delightful twist.

3. **Coconut-Lime Energy Bites**

Ingredients:

- 1 cup shredded coconut
- 1 cup cashews
- 1 cup dates, pitted
- Zest and juice of 2 limes
- Pinch of sea salt

Instructions:

1. **Blend Ingredients:**
   - In a food processor, blend shredded coconut, cashews, dates, lime zest, lime juice, and a pinch of sea salt until a sticky dough forms.

2. **Form Bites:**
   - Roll the mixture into bite-sized energy balls.

3. **Chill:**
   - Chill the coconut-lime energy bites in the refrigerator for at least 30 minutes.

4. **Serve:**
   - Serve these zesty energy bites for a refreshing and nutritious twist on dessert.

4. **Chai-Spiced Poached Pears**

Ingredients:

- 4 ripe but firm pears, peeled and halved
- 2 cups chai tea (brewed and cooled)
- 1/2 cup maple syrup
- 1 cinnamon stick
- 4 whole cloves
- 1 star anise

Instructions:

1. **Poach Pears:**
   - In a saucepan, combine chai tea, maple syrup, cinnamon stick, cloves, and star anise.
   - Once the pears are soft, add the halves and simmer.

2. **Cool:**
   - Let the poached pears cool in the liquid used to poach them.

3. **Serve:**
   - Serve the chai-spiced poached pears with a drizzle of the poaching liquid for a fragrant and sophisticated dessert twist.

5. **Pistachio-Rosewater Rice Pudding**

Ingredients:

- 1 cup arborio rice
- 4 cups coconut milk
- 1/2 cup sugar
- 1/2 cup pistachios, chopped
- 1 teaspoon rosewater
- Rose petals for garnish (optional)

Instructions:

1. **Cook Rice Pudding:**
   - In a saucepan, cook arborio rice with coconut milk and sugar until creamy and thickened.

2. **Add Pistachios and Rosewater:**
   - Stir in chopped pistachios and rosewater.

3. **Cool:**
   - Go ahead and let the rice pudding cool.

4. **Garnish:**
   - Garnish with rose petals for a visually stunning and fragrant twist on traditional rice pudding.

These desserts with a twist add unique flavors and ingredients to classic recipes, offering a delightful and unexpected experience for your taste buds. Enjoy the creative twists on traditional desserts!

SWEET AND NUTRIENTS-RICH TREATS

Certainly! Here are 5 sweet and nutrient-rich treats recipes with instructions.

1. **Dark Chocolate-Dipped Strawberries with Almonds**

Ingredients:

- Fresh strawberries
- Dark chocolate (70% cocoa or higher)
- Almonds, chopped

Instructions:

1. **Melt Chocolate:**
   - Melt dark chocolate in a heatproof bowl.

2. **Dip Strawberries:**
   - Dip each strawberry into the melted chocolate.

3. **Sprinkle with Almonds:**
   - Sprinkle chopped almonds over the chocolate-coated strawberries.

4. **Chill:**
   - Place the dipped strawberries in the refrigerator until the chocolate hardens.

5. **Enjoy:**

- Enjoy these antioxidant-rich, sweet treats with a
satisfying crunch.

2. **Frozen Banana Bites with Peanut Butter**

Ingredients:

- Bananas, sliced
- Peanut butter
- Dark chocolate (optional)
- Chopped nuts or coconut flakes (optional)

Instructions:

1. **Spread Peanut Butter:**
   - Toast the banana slices with peanut butter.

2. **Create Sandwiches:**
   - Make banana "sandwiches" by placing a second
banana slice on top.

3. **Freeze:**
   - Freeze the banana bites until solid.

4. **Optional Chocolate Coating:**
   - Optionally, melt dark chocolate and dip frozen
banana bites. Sprinkle with chopped nuts or
coconut flakes.

5. **Serve:**
   - Serve these nutrient-rich frozen banana bites for
a sweet and satisfying treat.

3. **Chia Seed Pudding Parfait**

Ingredients:

- Chia seeds
- Almond milk
- Maple syrup or agave nectar
- Mixed berries
- Granola

Instructions:

1. **Make Chia Seed Pudding:**
   - Mix chia seeds with almond milk and sweeten with maple syrup or agave nectar. Let it sit until it thickens.

2. **Layer with Berries and Granola:**
   - In a glass, layer chia seed pudding with mixed berries and granola.

3. **Repeat Layers:**
   - Layers should be repeated until the glass is full.

4. **Chill:**
   - Chill the parfait in the refrigerator until ready to serve.

5. **Enjoy:**
   - Enjoy this nutrient-rich chia seed pudding parfait as a delightful and guilt-free dessert.

4. **Fruit and Nut Energy Bites**

Ingredients:

- Dried apricots
- Dates, pitted
- Almonds
- Chia seeds
- Unsweetened shredded coconut

Instructions:

1. **Blend Ingredients:**
   - In a food processor, blend dried apricots, dates, almonds, and chia seeds until a sticky dough forms.

2. **Roll into Bites:**
   - Form the mixture into tiny bite-sized energy balls.

3. **Coat with Coconut:**
   - Roll the energy bites in unsweetened shredded coconut.

4. **Chill:**
   - Chill the fruit and nut energy bites in the refrigerator.

5. **Serve:**
   - Serve these nutrient-rich energy bites for a sweet and satisfying treat.

5. **Berry and Oat Breakfast Bars**

Ingredients:

- Rolled oats
- Mixed berries (fresh or frozen)
- Almond butter
- Maple syrup
- Chia seeds

Instructions:

1. **Mix Ingredients:**
   - Mix rolled oats, mixed berries, almond butter, maple syrup, and chia seeds in a bowl.

2. **Press into Bars:**
   - Press the mixture into a lined baking dish to form bars.

3. **Bake:**
   - Bake in the oven until the bars are firm and golden.

4. **Cool and Cut:**
   - Allow to cool fully before cutting into bars.

5. **Enjoy:**
   - Enjoy these nutrient-rich berry and oat breakfast bars as a wholesome and sweet treat.

These sweet and nutrient-rich treats offer a delicious way to satisfy your sweet tooth while providing essential nutrients. Enjoy these guilt-free options for a delightful and wholesome dessert experience!

FRUIT-BASED DESSERTS

Certainly! Here are 5 fruit-based desserts recipes with instructions.

1. **Mango Coconut Chia Pudding**

Ingredients:

- Chia seeds
- Coconut milk
- Mango, diced
- Maple syrup or agave nectar

Instructions:

1. **Make Chia Pudding:**
   - Mix chia seeds with coconut milk and sweeten with maple syrup or agave nectar. Let it get thicker in the fridge.

2. **Layer with Mango:**
   - Arrange the chopped mango on top of the chia pudding in serving glasses.

3. **Repeat Layers:**
   - Layers should be repeated until the glass is full.

4. **Chill:**
   - Chill the mango coconut chia pudding until ready to serve.

5. **Garnish:**
   - Garnish with additional diced mango for a tropical and refreshing fruit-based dessert.

2. **Grilled Pineapple with Cinnamon**

Ingredients:

- Pineapple slices
- Cinnamon powder
- Honey or maple syrup (optional)

Instructions:

1. **Grill Pineapple:**
   - Grill slices of pineapple until they get grill marks.

2. **Sprinkle with Cinnamon:**
   - Sprinkle grilled pineapple with cinnamon powder.

3. **Optional Sweetener:**
   - For extra sweetness, drizzle with maple syrup or honey.

4. **Serve:**
   - Serve this warm and spiced grilled pineapple for a simple and delightful fruit-based dessert.

3. **Mixed Berry Parfait**

Ingredients:

- Mixed berries (strawberries, blueberries, raspberries)
- Vegan yogurt or Greek yogurt
- Granola

Instructions:

1. **Layer with Berries:**
   - In a glass or bowl, layer mixed berries with vegan or Greek yogurt.

2. **Add Granola:**
   - Sprinkle granola over the berry and yogurt layers.

3. **Repeat Layers:**
   - Layers should be repeated until the glass is full.

4. **Garnish:**
   - Garnish the top with a few whole berries.

5. **Enjoy:**
   - Enjoy this refreshing and colorful mixed berry parfait as a light fruit-based dessert.

4. **Watermelon Mint Salad**

Ingredients:

- Watermelon, cubed
- Fresh mint leaves, chopped
- Lime juice

Instructions:

1. **Combine Watermelon and Mint:**
   - Toss cubed watermelon with chopped fresh mint leaves.

2. **Drizzle with Lime Juice:**
   - Drizzle lime juice over the watermelon and mint salad.

3. **Chill:**
   - Chill the watermelon mint salad for a refreshing and hydrating fruit-based dessert.

4. **Serve:**
   - Serve in bowls or as individual portions for a light and flavorful treat.

5. **Citrus Salad with Honey-Lime Dressing**

Ingredients:

- Orange segments

- Grapefruit segments
- Kiwi, sliced
- Honey-lime dressing (honey or maple syrup, lime juice)

Instructions:

1. **Arrange Citrus Fruits:**
   - Arrange orange and grapefruit segments along with sliced kiwi on a serving platter.

2. **Prepare Dressing:**
   - Whisk together honey or maple syrup with lime juice to create a sweet and tangy dressing.

3. **Drizzle Dressing:**
   - Drizzle the honey-lime dressing over the citrus fruit salad.

4. **Chill:**
   - Chill the citrus salad before serving for a cool and citrusy fruit-based dessert.

5. **Garnish:**
   - For extra freshness, sprinkle some fresh mint leaves on top.

These fruit-based desserts showcase the natural sweetness and vibrant colors of various fruits, making them a healthy and delightful choice for satisfying your sweet cravings. Enjoy the freshness of these delicious treats!

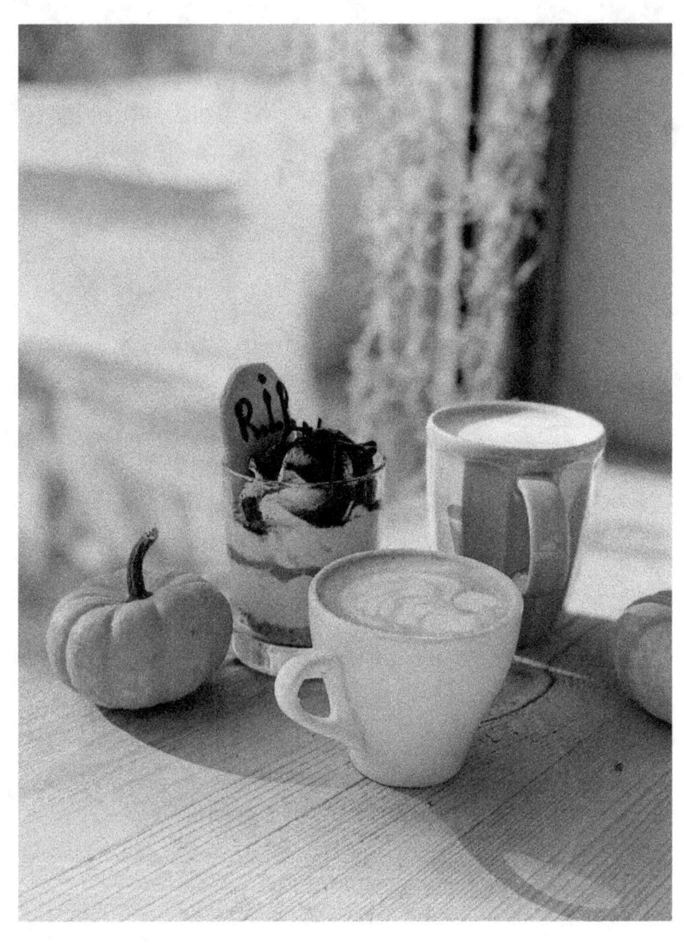

CHAPTER EIGHT

MEAL PREP AND PLANNING

Meal Prep and Planning Guide

1. Set Your Goals:
   - Define your nutritional goals, dietary preferences, and portion sizes to guide your meal planning.

2. Choose a Meal Prep Day:
   - Designate a specific day each week for meal prep to streamline the process.

3. Create a Weekly Menu:
   - Plan your meals for the week, considering a balance of proteins, carbohydrates, and healthy fats.

4. Make a Shopping List:
   - Based on your weekly menu, create a detailed shopping list to avoid unnecessary trips to the grocery store.

5. Batch Cooking:
   - Cook large quantities of staples like grains, proteins, and roasted vegetables to use in multiple meals.

6. Portion Control:

- Use portion control containers or labels to ensure balanced servings for each meal.

7. Variety is Key:
   - Incorporate a variety of colors, textures, and flavors to keep your meals interesting and nutritionally diverse.

8. Cook Once, Eat Twice:
   - Repurpose ingredients to create new meals throughout the week, reducing cooking time.

9. Invest in Quality Containers:
   - Use durable, airtight containers to store and transport your meals safely.

10. Include Snacks:
   - Plan and prep healthy snacks like cut fruits, vegetable sticks, or energy bites to curb cravings.

11. Consider Freezing:
   - Freeze portions of meals that may not stay fresh for the entire week to minimize food waste.

12. Prep Breakfasts and Lunches:
   - Prioritize prepping breakfasts and lunches for convenience during busy mornings.

13. Mindful Labeling:
   - Label containers with the date of preparation to ensure freshness.

14. Hydration Planning:
   - Include water and hydrating beverages in your meal planning to stay adequately hydrated.

15. Schedule Time for Prep:
   - Allocate a specific time on your chosen meal prep day to focus on planning, shopping, and cooking.

16. Embrace Leftovers:
   - Embrace the concept of leftovers as a time-saving strategy, making use of cooked components in new dishes.

17. Try Theme Nights:
   - Incorporate theme nights (e.g., Meatless Monday, Taco Tuesday) to add excitement and structure to your meal plan.

18. Be Flexible:
   - Remain flexible and open to adjustments based on your schedule and preferences.

19. Review and Adjust:
   - Regularly review your meal prep routine and adjust as needed to keep it efficient and enjoyable.

20. Celebrate Success:
   - Acknowledge and celebrate your commitment to meal prep, recognizing the positive impact on your health and time management.

Consistent meal prep and planning contribute to a healthier lifestyle by saving time, reducing stress, and promoting mindful eating. Tailor these tips to fit your preferences and enjoy the benefits of organized and nutritious meals.

BATCH COOKING STRATEGIES

Batch Cooking Strategies for Efficient Meal Prep

1. Choose Versatile Ingredients:
   - Opt for versatile ingredients that can be used in multiple recipes to maximize efficiency.

2. Plan a Weekly Menu:
   - Create a weekly menu that incorporates batch-cooked ingredients into different meals.

3. Batch Cook Proteins:
   - Cook a large batch of proteins (chicken, tofu, beans) and use them in various dishes like salads, wraps, and stir-fries.

4. Roast Vegetables in Batches:
   - Roast a variety of vegetables in large quantities and use them as sides, in grain bowls, or as toppings for salads.

5. Make Big Batches of Grains:

- Cook a large batch of grains (quinoa, brown rice, etc.) to use as a base for different meals throughout the week.

6. Utilize Slow Cookers and Instant Pots:
- Use slow cookers or Instant Pots to effortlessly prepare large batches of soups, stews, or chili.

7. Prep Snack Packs:
- Create snack packs with cut fruits, veggies, and nuts to have quick, grab-and-go snacks on hand.

8. Portion and Freeze:
- Portion meals into freezer-safe containers and freeze for future use, reducing the need for frequent cooking.

9. Incorporate Make-Ahead Sauces:
- Prepare sauces and dressings in advance to add flavor to meals without extra prep time.

10. Label and Date:
- Label and date each batch-cooked item to keep track of freshness and avoid food waste.

11. Cook in Stages:
- Break down your batch cooking into stages throughout the week for a more manageable process.

12. Theme Nights:

- Designate certain nights for specific cuisines (e.g., Italian, Mexican) to streamline ingredient preparation.

13. Repurpose Leftovers:
  - Be creative in repurposing leftovers into new dishes to keep meals interesting.

14. Efficient Storage:
  - Invest in a variety of storage containers, including portion-sized ones, to keep batch-cooked items organized.

15. Share the Load:
  - If possible, batch cook with family or friends to share the workload and exchange a variety of dishes.

16. Plan for Breakfast and Lunch:
  - Batch cook breakfast items like overnight oats or lunch options to streamline your morning routine.

17. Pre-Chop Ingredients:
  - Pre-chop vegetables, fruits, and herbs at the beginning of the week to save time during meal prep.

18. Monitor Inventory:
  - Regularly check your freezer and pantry to stay aware of batch-cooked items available for use.

19. Keep It Simple:

- Focus on a few key recipes each week to keep batch cooking manageable and enjoyable.

20. Celebrate Success:
   - Acknowledge the time and effort saved by batch cooking and celebrate the positive impact on your routine.

Batch cooking is a powerful strategy for efficient meal prep, saving time and ensuring you have nourishing meals readily available. Customize these strategies to fit your preferences and enjoy the benefits of a well-organized kitchen routine.

TIPS FOR EATING PLANT-BASED ON THE GO

Tips for Eating Plant-Based On the Go

1. **Plan Ahead:
   - Research and identify plant-based options at local restaurants or cafes before heading out.

2. **Pack Snacks:
   - Carry portable plant-based snacks like nuts, seeds, dried fruits, and energy bars for quick and convenient munching.

3. **Prep Quick Meals:

- Prepare easy-to-assemble meals, such as salads in a jar or wraps with hummus and veggies, that can be quickly put together.

4. **Explore Local Grocery Stores:
   - Visit local grocery stores or markets for fresh fruits, veggies, and other plant-based snacks that can be enjoyed on the go.

5. **Choose Plant-Based Restaurants:
   - Look for plant-based or vegetarian restaurants in the area to simplify your meal choices.

6. **Bring a Reusable Water Bottle:
   - Reusable water bottles can help you stay hydrated. To enhance the flavor, include cucumber or lemon slices.

7. **Research Chain Restaurant Menus:
   - Check the menus of chain restaurants; many offer plant-based options or can customize meals to your preference.

8. **BYO Container:
   - Bring your own container for takeout to minimize waste and ensure you have a suitable vessel for leftovers.

9. **Learn Basic Ingredient Substitutions:
   - Familiarize yourself with basic ingredient substitutions to modify non-plant-based dishes into plant-based ones.

10. **Pack a Portable Lunch Cooler:
   - Invest in a small cooler to carry perishable items like salads, sandwiches, or fruit without compromising freshness.

11. **Stock Up on Non-Perishables:
   - Keep non-perishable plant-based items in your bag, such as whole-grain crackers, nut butter packets, or instant soup cups.

12. **Choose Whole Fruits:
   - Opt for whole fruits like apples, bananas, or oranges that are easy to carry and require minimal preparation.

13. **Find Salad Bars or Buffets:
   - Locate restaurants with salad bars or buffets, allowing you to choose a variety of plant-based options.

14. **Use Food Delivery Services:
   - Explore food delivery apps that offer plant-based restaurant options delivered to your location.

15. **Learn Local Cuisine:
   - Learn about the local cuisine at your destination and identify plant-based dishes that are part of the culinary tradition.

16. **Create DIY Trail Mix:

- Mix nuts, seeds, dried fruits, and a touch of dark chocolate to create your own plant-based trail mix for a quick and satisfying snack.

17. **Master the Art of the Veggie Bowl:
   - Order or create veggie bowls with a mix of grains, beans, veggies, and a tasty sauce for a filling and nutritious on-the-go meal.

18. **Seek Out Smoothie or Juice Bars:
   - Look for smoothie or juice bars that offer plant-based options loaded with fruits, vegetables, and plant-based protein.

19. **Stay Informed About Local Ingredients:
   - Familiarize yourself with local plant-based ingredients that can be easily incorporated into meals or snacks.

20. **Embrace Convenience Stores:
   - Many convenience stores offer plant-based options like fresh fruit, nuts, and plant-based snacks—check their selection.

Eating plant-based on the go is achievable with a bit of planning and creativity. These tips can help you maintain a plant-based lifestyle while navigating a busy schedule or traveling.

CHAPTER NINE

FITNESS AND NUTRITION TIPS

The following are some fitness and nutrition tips for
a healthy lifestyle

1. **Balanced Diet:
   - Prioritize a balanced diet with a variety of fruits,
vegetables, whole grains, lean proteins, and
healthy fats.

2. **Stay Hydrated:
   - Throughout the day, sip a sufficient amount of
water to maintain your hydration and general
wellbeing.

3. **Portion Control:
   - Pay attention to portion proportions to prevent
overindulging and to keep your weight in check.

4. **Incorporate Plant-Based Meals:
   - Include plant-based meals to increase fiber
intake and benefit from a variety of nutrients.

5. **Prep Healthy Snacks:
   - Prepare nutrient-dense snacks like cut
vegetables, fruit, or homemade energy bites to curb
unhealthy cravings.

6. **Prioritize Protein:

- Ensure you get enough protein from sources like beans, lentils, tofu, and lean plant-based proteins.

7. **Choose Whole Foods:
- Opt for whole, minimally processed foods over heavily processed options for better nutrition.

8. **Meal Timing:
- Consider meal timing to support energy levels, such as having a balanced meal before a workout.

9. **Mindful Eating:
- Savor each bite and be aware of your body's signals of hunger and fullness to engage in mindful eating.

10. **Variety is Key:
- Eat a variety of colors and types of food to ensure a broad range of nutrients in your diet.

11. **Regular Exercise:
- Incorporate regular physical activity into your routine, including a mix of cardio, strength training, and flexibility exercises.

12. **Set Realistic Goals:
- Set achievable fitness and nutrition goals that align with your lifestyle and preferences.

13. **Meal Prep:

- Plan and prepare meals in advance to make healthier choices and save time during busy days.

14. **Limit Added Sugars:
- Reduce consumption of foods and beverages high in added sugars to promote better overall health.

15. **Listen to Your Body:
- Pay attention to your body's signals for hunger, fullness, and fatigue to make informed decisions about eating and exercise.

16. **Prioritize Sleep:
- Ensure adequate and quality sleep as it plays a crucial role in overall health, including weight management.

17. **Supplement Wisely:
- If needed, consult with a healthcare professional to determine if supplements, such as vitamin B12 or omega-3s, are necessary for your diet.

18. **Mind-Body Connection:
- Explore mind-body activities like yoga or meditation to promote mental well-being and stress reduction.

19. **Celebrate Progress:
- Celebrate small victories and progress on your fitness and nutrition journey to stay motivated.

20. **Stay Informed:
  - Stay informed about nutrition trends and exercise techniques to continually enhance your health knowledge.

Adopting a combination of balanced nutrition and regular physical activity contributes to a healthy and sustainable lifestyle. These tips can help you create habits that support your overall well-being.

PLANT-BASED NUTRITION FOR ACTIVE LIFESTYLE

Plant-Based Nutrition for an Active Lifestyle

1. **Adequate Protein Intake:
  - Incorporate plant-based protein sources such as beans, lentils, tofu, tempeh, quinoa, and edamame to support muscle recovery and growth.

2. **Whole Grains for Energy:
  - Choose whole grains like brown rice, quinoa, oats, and whole wheat for sustained energy during workouts.

3. **Healthy Fats:
  - Include sources of healthy fats like avocados, nuts, seeds, and olive oil for overall health and energy.

4. **Hydration with Plant-Based Beverages:

  - Stay hydrated with water, herbal teas, or plant-based milk alternatives like almond, soy, or oat milk.

5. **Nutrient-Dense Snacking:
  - Snack on nutrient-dense options such as raw nuts, seeds, fresh fruit, or vegetable sticks for sustained energy throughout the day.

6. **Pre-Workout Fuel:
  - Have a balanced pre-workout meal with a mix of carbohydrates and a moderate amount of protein for energy and muscle support.

7. **Post-Workout Recovery:
  - Opt for a post-workout meal or snack that includes a combination of carbohydrates and plant-based protein for recovery.

8. **Leafy Greens and Iron-Rich Foods:
  - Consume leafy greens, lentils, beans, and fortified cereals for iron, which is essential for oxygen transport during physical activity.

9. **Omega-3 Fatty Acids:
  - Include plant-based sources of omega-3 fatty acids like chia seeds, flaxseeds, walnuts, and hemp seeds for anti-inflammatory benefits.

10. **Vitamin B12 Supplementation:

- Consider a vitamin B12 supplement, as it is primarily found in animal products. Seek the counsel of a medical expert for tailored guidance.

11. **Calcium-Rich Plant Foods:
  - Ensure an adequate intake of calcium from plant sources like fortified plant milk, tofu, kale, and almonds for bone health.

12. **Antioxidant-Rich Foods:
  - Incorporate fruits and vegetables with vibrant colors to benefit from antioxidants that aid in recovery and immune function.

13. **Plant-Based Protein Shakes:
  - Consider plant-based protein shakes made with ingredients like pea, hemp, or rice protein for a convenient post-workout option.

14. **Meal Timing:
  - Pay attention to meal timing, having a balanced meal or snack 2-3 hours before exercising and a post-workout meal within an hour after.

15. **Variety in Plant-Based Proteins:
  - Mix up your protein sources to ensure a diverse amino acid profile. Combine legumes, grains, and seeds throughout the day.

16. **Electrolyte-Rich Foods:

- Consume electrolyte-rich foods like bananas, oranges, and potatoes to replenish minerals lost through sweat during exercise.

17. **Mindful Eating Practices:
   - Practice mindful eating to listen to your body's hunger and fullness cues, supporting optimal fueling for your activity level.

18. **Experiment with Plant-Based Recipes:
   - Explore and experiment with plant-based recipes to keep your meals exciting and enjoyable.

19. **Consult a Registered Dietitian:
   - If needed, consult with a registered dietitian who specializes in plant-based nutrition to ensure you meet your specific dietary needs.

20. **Balanced Macros and Micros:
   - Aim for a balance of macronutrients (carbohydrates, proteins, fats) and micronutrients (vitamins and minerals) for overall health and performance.

Adopting a plant-based diet for an active lifestyle requires thoughtful planning to ensure you receive adequate nutrients for energy, recovery, and overall well-being. Customize your plant-based nutrition to meet your individual needs and consult with a healthcare professional or registered dietitian for personalized advice.

INCORPORATING PLANT-BASED EATING IN TO WORKOUT ROUTINES

Incorporating Plant-Based Eating into Workout Routines

1. **Pre-Workout Fuel:
   - Consume a balanced pre-workout meal containing complex carbohydrates (whole grains, fruits) and plant-based protein (legumes, tofu) for sustained energy.

2. **Hydration with Plant-Based Options:
   - Stay hydrated with water, coconut water, or herbal teas. Electrolyte-rich drinks can be homemade using plant-based ingredients.

3. **Smoothies and Protein Shakes:
   - Include plant-based smoothies or protein shakes with ingredients like fruits, leafy greens, plant-based protein powders, and nut butter for a quick and convenient pre or post-workout option.

4. **Snack Smart:
   - Have nutrient-dense snacks like a handful of nuts, a piece of fruit, or whole-grain crackers with hummus between meals to maintain energy levels.

5. **Post-Workout Recovery:
   - Opt for a post-workout meal or snack that combines carbohydrates and plant-based protein to

aid in muscle recovery. Examples include a quinoa bowl with veggies and tofu or a lentil-based soup.

6. **Whole Foods for Nutrient Density:
   - Choose whole, minimally processed foods for their nutrient density. Throughout your meals, include a range of fruits, vegetables, whole grains, and legumes.

7. **Protein-Packed Meals:
   - Plan meals that feature plant-based protein sources such as beans, lentils, chickpeas, tempeh, and edamame. Include a variety of these proteins throughout the day.

8. **Antioxidant-Rich Foods:
   - Consume antioxidant-rich foods like berries, dark leafy greens, and nuts to help combat oxidative stress that may occur during intense workouts.

9. **Experiment with Plant-Based Recipes:
   - Keep your meals interesting by experimenting with a variety of plant-based recipes. This can help prevent boredom and ensure you get a diverse range of nutrients.

10. **Balanced Nutrient Timing:
   - Pay attention to nutrient timing. Consume a combination of carbohydrates and protein within a reasonable time frame after your workout to support recovery.

11. **Plant-Based Protein Sources:
   - Diversify your plant-based protein sources to ensure a complete amino acid profile. Combine and contrast grains, seeds, nuts, and legumes.

12. **Incorporate Whole Grains:
   - Choose whole grains such as quinoa, brown rice, and oats for their complex carbohydrates, providing a steady release of energy.

13. **Recovery Smoothies:
   - Create recovery smoothies with ingredients like almond milk, frozen berries, banana, and a scoop of plant-based protein powder for a delicious and nutrient-packed option.

14. **Protein-Rich Snacks:
   - Keep protein-rich snacks handy, such as roasted chickpeas, edamame, or a small serving of hummus with veggies.

15. **Mindful Eating Practices:
   - Practice mindful eating to connect with your body's hunger and fullness cues, promoting a balanced and intuitive approach to fueling your workouts.

16. **Plan and Prep:
   - Plan and prep your meals in advance to ensure that you have plant-based options readily available, especially during busy days.

17. **Stay Hydrated:
   - Hydrate before, during, and after your workout.
Fruits and vegetables high in water content might
help you stay hydrated overall.

18. **Listen to Your Body:**
   - Observe your reactions to various foods and
modify your diet accordingly. Listening to your body
is key to optimizing your performance.

19. **Consult with a Professional:**
   - If needed, consult with a registered dietitian or
nutritionist who specializes in plant-based nutrition
for personalized guidance tailored to your specific
workout routine and goals.

Incorporating plant-based eating into your workout
routine requires thoughtful planning to ensure you
meet your nutritional needs for energy, recovery,
and performance. Customize your plant-based
nutrition plan based on your individual preferences,
dietary requirements, and workout intensity.

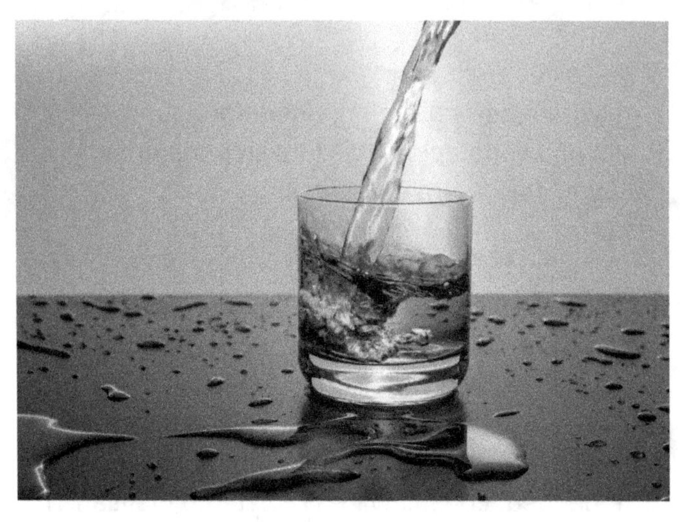

CONCLUSION

Conclusion: Embracing a Plant-Powered Lifestyle

In concluding this journey through the realms of plant-based living, we've explored the diverse chapters of a lifestyle that goes beyond mere dietary choices—it's a holistic embrace of well-being, compassion, and sustainability. From the tantalizing flavors of nutrient-rich dishes to the rhythmic beat of workout routines, the plant-based lifestyle offers a symphony of benefits.

Plant-Based Nutrition Unveiled:
  - We uncovered the vibrant tapestry of plant-based nutrition, exploring essential ingredients, protein sources, whole grains, and nutritional powerhouses in the form of vegetables and fruits. The kitchen transformed into a realm of culinary creativity, guided by flavorful seasonings and essential kitchen tools and techniques.

Plant-Based Morning Rituals:
  - Breakfasts for champions unfolded in a feast of protein-packed smoothie bowls, hearty oatmeal variations, and energizing breakfast burritos, providing the perfect start to active days.

Power-Packed Lunches and Colorful Salads:
  - Midday adventures introduced us to power-packed lunches, colorful salad bowls,

protein-rich sandwiches and wraps, and hearty grain bowls—all celebrating the versatility of plant-based ingredients.

Muscle-Building Dinners and Wholesome Combos:
  - As the sun set, muscle-building dinners took center stage with plant-based protein main courses, wholesome grain and vegetable combos, and comforting one-pot meals that tantalize the taste buds and nourish the body.

Snack Innovations and Guilt-Free Indulgences:
  - The snack attack unfolded with nut and seed mixes, guilt-free chips and dips, and creative plant-based snack ideas—showcasing that indulgence can be both delicious and nutritious.

Desserts with a Twist and Sweet Treats:
  - Dessert wasn't forgotten as we explored desserts with a twist, sweet and nutrient-rich treats, and fruit-based delights—proving that the plant-based palette extends to the realm of satisfying sweetness.

Mastering Meal Prep and Planning:
  - The journey continued with insights into meal prep and planning, unveiling batch cooking strategies and offering sample weekly meal plans—a testament to the practicality and sustainability of a plant-based lifestyle.

Fitness and Nutrition Synergy:
   - Fitness and nutrition became steadfast companions, with tips for eating plant-based on the go and strategies for incorporating plant-based eating into workout routines. The connection between a plant-based diet and enhanced fitness performance became evident.

Plant-Powered Success Stories:
   - Finally, we delved into inspiring success stories and testimonies, where individuals discovered not only the physical benefits of a plant-based lifestyle but also the profound impact on mental well-being, relationships, and a sense of connection to the broader community.

In conclusion, the journey through plant-based living unveils a pathway to a life filled with vibrant health, ethical choices, and culinary delights. It's an invitation to savor the richness of plant-based nutrition, embrace the energy of active living, and bask in the stories of those who have discovered the transformative power of plants.

As you embark on or continue your plant-powered journey, may each plant-based meal be a celebration of health, sustainability, and joy. Here's to a thriving life, rooted in the nourishment of plants.

FINAL TIPS AND ENCOURAGEMENT

Final Tips and Encouragement for Your Plant-Powered Journey

1. **Start Small, Go at Your Pace:
   - Begin by incorporating one plant-based meal at a time. Gradually experiment with new recipes and ingredients at your own pace.

2. **Explore Diverse Flavors:
   - Embrace the rich tapestry of plant-based flavors. Experiment with herbs, spices, and unique ingredients to keep your meals exciting and satisfying.

3. **Listen to Your Body:
   - Take note of your feelings after eating various foods. Your body is an excellent guide, so listen to its cues and adjust your plant-based choices accordingly.

4. **Connect with the Community:
   - Join online forums, social media groups, or local plant-based meet-ups to connect with others on a similar journey. Sharing experiences and tips can be both inspiring and supportive.

5. **Plan and Prep Ahead:

- Meal preparation and planning ahead of time can change everything. It not only saves time but ensures you have nutritious plant-based options readily available.

6. **Stay Educated:
   - Keep yourself informed about plant-based nutrition, cooking techniques, and the latest recipes. The more you know, the more confidently you can navigate your plant-powered lifestyle.

7. **Celebrate Progress, Not Perfection:
   - Celebrate your successes, big and small. Recall that adopting a plant-based diet is a journey rather than a destination. Progress is what matters.

8. **Involve Family and Friends:
   - Share the joy of plant-based eating with your loved ones. Involve them in cooking, introduce them to new flavors, and make it a positive, shared experience.

9. **Variety is Key:
   - Keep your meals diverse by incorporating a wide range of fruits, vegetables, grains, and proteins. This guarantees that you receive a wide range of nutrients.

10. **Be Mindful of Nutrient Needs:
   - Pay attention to essential nutrients like B12, iron, calcium, and omega-3s. Consider

supplements or fortified foods to meet these needs
if necessary.

11. **Enjoy the Journey:
   - Accept the adventure of trying out new dishes
and flavors. Plant-based eating isn't a restriction;
it's an exploration of a world of culinary possibilities.

12. **Balance and Moderation:
   - Aim for balance and moderation in your
plant-based choices. A well-rounded diet with a
variety of nutrients is the key to sustained
well-being.

13. **Stay Positive in Social Settings:
   - Approach social situations with a positive
mindset. Communicate your dietary choices calmly,
and don't be afraid to bring a dish to share at
gatherings.

14. **Mindful Eating Practices:
   - Practice mindful eating by savoring each bite,
eating slowly, and appreciating the nourishment
your food provides.

15. **Explore Local and Seasonal Produce:
   - Encourage your local producers and look at
seasonal foods. It not only benefits the environment
but introduces you to fresh, local flavors.

16. **Cook with Love:

- Infuse your plant-based meals with love and intention. Cooking becomes a joyful act when you appreciate the nourishment you're providing for yourself.

17. **Be Adventurous:
   - Don't shy away from trying new foods and recipes. The plant-based world is vast, and there's always something new to discover.

18. **Share Your Journey:
   - Share your plant-powered journey with others. Your experiences and successes may inspire those around you to explore the benefits of a plant-based lifestyle.

19. **Embrace Imperfection:
   - Understand that not every meal needs to be perfect, and there will be times when convenience takes precedence. Embrace the imperfections and continue learning.

20. **Remember Your "Why":
   - Reflect on the reasons that led you to embrace a plant-based lifestyle. Whether for health, environmental, or ethical reasons, reconnecting with your "why" can be a powerful motivator.

As you navigate the vibrant landscape of plant-based living, may these tips serve as guiding lights on your journey. Embrace the joy of nourishing yourself with plant-powered goodness, and may your path be filled with health, vitality, and the satisfaction of making choices that align with your well-being and values. Here's to your continued success on your plant-powered adventure!